Objective Structured Clinical Examination

in

Intensive
Care
Medicine

Jeyasankar Jeyanathan Daniel Owens

tfm Publishing Limited, Castle Hill Barns, Harley, Shrewsbury, SY5 6LX, UK
Tel: +44 (0)1952 510061; Fax: +44 (0)1952 510192
E-mail: info@tfmpublishing.com
Web site: www.tfmpublishing.com

Editing, design & typesetting: Nikki Bramhill BSc Hons Dip Law
First edition: © 2016

Paperback	ISBN:	978-1-910079-23-2
E-book editions:	2016	
ePub	ISBN:	978-1-910079-24-9
Mobi	ISBN:	978-1-910079-25-6
Web pdf	ISBN:	978-1-910079-26-3

Printed by Cambrian Printers, Llanbadarn Road, Aberystwyth, Ceredigion, SY23 3TN
Tel: +44 (0)1970 627111; Web site: www.cambrian-printers.co.uk

Contents

Chapter 3

Chapter 4

Chapter 5

Index

Preface

Objective Structured Clinical Examinations (OSCEs) in medicine are not a new phenomenon. Intensive care exams across the world are now incorporating this form of examination as part of the assessment process. Take for example the Fellowship of the Faculty of Intensive Care Medicine (FFICM) examination in the United Kingdom (UK) which now includes OSCEs; thus, they are gaining further importance.

There are a number of intensive care medicine (ICM) textbooks available, but there are very few resources specifically aimed at the practice of OSCEs in ICM. This book is not designed to be a textbook; rather, it has been specifically designed to implement the rehearsal of OSCEs. Much like a driving test there are certain things in the OSCEs that must be said to score that ever precious mark, even if it is stating the absolute obvious, for example:

This is a critical emergency and I would undertake:

• An acute assessment, resuscitation and management to follow an 'airway, breathing, circulation, disability and exposure' approach.

Small and compact in design, this book can be utilised for practice in the immediate days running up to an ICM exam. Previous exam topic favourites have been carefully analysed before the preparation of this book. It will aid the reader to polish their OSCE performance and possibly identify areas that may have been neglected.

Depending on the exam that you will sit, a fair proportion of questions will require answers in the form of lists (e.g. list of tests you would order). In our experience this often leads to the examiner repeating the phrase "anything else?"! Try not to get thrown by this; you may have given an excellent answer but there is still a further mark for the one thing you didn't mention and the examiner is trying to give you the opportunity to score that final mark! No matter how good your knowledge is, everyone forgets something in the heat of the exam! The OSCE answers and narratives in the book have been purposely arranged as bulleted lists timed for 6-minute stations. This is because every station in an OSCE exam has listed scoring marks which are available in that finite time of 6 minutes. With practice, your 'OSCE mindset' can be arranged so as to score marks in a systematic and organised, yet swift, manner. For example, in this chest X-ray, what are some of the causes of bilateral pulmonary infiltrates?:

- Pulmonary oedema:
  - cardiac failure;
  - valvular heart disease — congenital or acquired;
  - renal failure;
  - liver failure;
  - iatrogenic fluid overload.
- Infection:
  - bacterial;
  - viral;
  - fungal or protozoal;
- Autoimmune:
  - Goodpasture's syndrome;
  - pulmonary fibrosis.
- Acute respiratory distress syndrome (ARDS).

(4 marks — 1 mark for each correct main stem with appropriate sub-stem examples.)

Your brain should 'sieve' out the useful information in these situations, to ensure that you are at least scoring marks in different organ systems. In this example, it is entirely possible to state "ARDS" and "pulmonary oedema", and then waste precious time trying to state causes in a haphazard manner. The practice of answering as an organised bulleted list allows important marks to be scored, whilst saving time to pick up further marks in other subsequent questions.

Scoring systems have come up in past OSCE exams, hence many of the important ones have been incorporated into the chapters.

Remember that if you are sitting an exam with a viva element, there is the possibility of topic cross-over from the OSCE to the viva and vice versa. To that aim, when using this book, it is worth trying to outline how you would answer the OSCE topic were you given it in a viva setting.

Simulation stations can form a station in ICM OSCEs. We have made a conscious decision not to include them in the OSCE sets presented here, as high-fidelity simulation is very difficult to emulate through a book. Instead we have provided additional stations which could well form the basis of a simulation station.

We have included 'Top Tip' boxes to provide clues as to what the examiners are looking for and what they are expecting from your answers. These tips have been assembled from the principal knowledge and experience of candidates who have undertaken ICM exams, hence they are well worth noting.

You will be examined in at least one of the so-called 'professionalism' stations, colloquially referred to as 'communication skills' stations, during the examination. Commonly, these involve the use of actors, rather than patients, and you need to develop a strategy for dealing with the 'method' actor who takes their role too seriously. Colleagues of ours have often expressed frustration when the 'daughter' of the simulated patient spent so much time crying that it proved very difficult to progress with the station. Unfortunately, we have no magic formula for this occurrence, but highlighting the possibility of it happening will give you an opportunity to try to work out a strategy to deal with this. The professionalism stations we have included in this book do often read a little like a list; unfortunately, we can't find any other way of introducing these types of topics. You will need to rely on your 'sparring partner' to embellish these stations into something that resembles the OSCE station. The station gives you the topic and a standard marking scheme but you will need a colleague to role play the actor's part.

It is not uncommon for the same or similar topics to come up in the same exam, especially if they are deemed important, though as question banks increase in size this is less of an issue. If it does happen make sure you listen in case the focus of the question is different, and be thankful.

There are a number of more 'formulaic' stations and we have attempted to provide a system to answer these. The most common of these is the dreaded electrocardiogram (ECG) station. Our advice would be to decide on your system of interpreting and presenting an ECG (we've outlined one very simple method in the book). Even if you have no idea what the ECG shows, you will be at least scoring marks as you go through it systematically. When presented with the next ECG do the same; the examiner will most likely tell you if they do not want you to do this again, in which case if you don't know the diagnosis you will struggle. In our conversations with examiners, there are often marks for this systematic approach, so don't miss out.

This is unlikely to be the first OSCE that you have sat in your medical career, so remember that all the rules you learnt at medical school still apply. If you have a bad station, forget it and move on. If you don't know the answer to a question and the examiner is failing to move on then tell them! Most stations are designed to allow you to score marks, even if you fail to score the mark for the diagnosis.

Whilst both authors have been through the UK intensive care training programme, we have tried hard to minimise any possible bias towards examinations in the UK and Europe, in order to achieve a more global appeal. Thus, the book is relevant for any ICM examination that contains an OSCE element. For those of you taking European-based exams, we have had contact with examiners for the European Diploma in Intensive Care Medicine (EDIC), as well as the newly created Fellowship of the Faculty of Intensive Care Medicine (FFICM) in the UK. Many of these stations are based on real topics which have come up in both of these two examinations over the last few years; however, we have been careful to try and remove any European eccentricities, especially with respect to acronyms! As such we are confident that this book will prove an excellent training tool for any ICM exam which employs the OSCE format.

We wish you the best of luck with the exam you are about to take and look forward to seeing well-thumbed copies of this book on the nurses' station in intensive care units (ICUs) across the country! We want the book to be a resource for colleagues to hone their skills for an OSCE format. The book should be the perfect way of packing in 10 minutes of OSCE revision before the next ICU ward round starts!

Jeyasankar Jeyanathan BMedSci (Hons) MBBS DMCC Pgcert (Med Sim) FRCA FFICM
Daniel Owens BSc (Hons) MBBS Pgcert (Med Ed) FRCA FFICM
Intensive Care Unit, St George's Hospital, London, UK

Abbreviations

ABG	Arterial blood gas
Ach	Acetylcholine
ACS	Abdominal compartment syndrome
ACTH	Adrenocorticotropic hormone
ADH	Antidiuretic hormone
AF	Atrial fibrillation
AFB	Acid-fast bacillus
AKI	Acute kidney injury
ALP	Alkaline phosphatase
ALT	Alanine aminotransferase
AMTS	Abbreviated Mental Test Score
AP	Anteroposterior
aPTT	Activated partial thromboplastin time
ARDS	Acute respiratory distress syndrome
AST	Aspartate aminotransferase
AVN	Atrioventricular node
BAL	Broncho-alveolar lavage
BC	Blood culture
BDS	British Diabetes Society
BE	Base excess
BMI	Body mass index
BNP	B-natriuretic peptide
BP	Blood pressure
BTS	British Thoracic Society
Ca	Calcium
CAM-ICU	Confusion Assessment Method for the Intensive Care Unit
CAP	Community-acquired pneumonia
CCF	Congestive cardiac failure
CCS	Corticosteroid
CI	Cardiac index
CK	Creatine kinase
Cl⁻	Chloride

cmH_2O	Centimetres of water
CMV	*Cytomegalovirus*
CO_2	Carbon dioxide
CO	Cardiac output
COPD	Chronic obstructive pulmonary disease
CPAP	Continuous positive airway pressure
CPP	Cerebral perfusion pressure
CPR	Cardiopulmonary resuscitation
CRP	C-reactive protein
CSF	Cerebrospinal fluid
CSWS	Cerebral salt wasting syndrome
CT	Computed tomography
CVA	Cerebrovascular event
CVP	Central venous pressure
CVVDF	Continuous veno-venous diafiltration
CVVHDF	Continuous veno-venous haemodiafiltration
CVVHF	Continuous veno-venous haemofiltration
CXR	Chest X-ray
DDAVP	Desmopressin
DI	Diabetes insipidus
DIC	Disseminated intravascular coagulation
DKA	Diabetic ketoacidosis
DO_2I	Oxygen delivery index
DVT	Deep vein thrombosis
EBV	Ebstein-Barr virus
ECG	Electrocardiogram
ECMO	Extracorporeal membrane oxygenation
EGDT	Early goal-directed therapy
ELISA	Enzyme-linked immunosorbent assay
ERCP	Endoscopic retrograde cholangiopancreatography
ESR	Erythrocyte sedimentation rate
$ETCO_2$	End-tidal carbon dioxide
ETT	Endotracheal tube
EVD	External ventricular drain
FBC	Full blood count
FFP	Fresh frozen plasma
FIB	Fascia iliaca block
FiO_2	Fractional concentration of inspired oxygen

FRC	Functional residual capacity
GCS	Glasgow Coma Scale
GGT	Gamma-glutamyl transpeptidase
GI	Gastrointestinal
GTN	Glyceryl trinitrate
Hb	Haemoglobin
HES	Hydroxyethyl starch
HFOV	High-frequency oscillatory ventilation
HHS	Hyperglycaemic hyperosmolar state
HITTS	Heparin-induced thrombotic thrombocytopenic syndrome
HR	Heart rate
HTLV	Human T-cell lymphotrophic virus
IABP	Invasive arterial blood pressure
IABP	Intra-aortic balloon pump
IAH	Intra-abdominal hypertension
IAP	Intra-abdominal pressure
ICM	Intensive care medicine
ICP	Intracranial pressure
ICU	Intensive care unit
IE	Infective endocarditis
INR	International Normalised Ratio
IV	Intravenous
IVDU	Intravenous drug use
IVIg	Intravenous immunoglobulin
K^+	Potassium
kPa	Kilo Pascals
LA	Local anaesthetic
LBBB	Left bundle branch block
LDH	Lactate dehydrogenase
LFT	Liver function test
LIDCO	Lithium dilution cardiac output monitoring
LMWH	Low-molecular-weight heparin
LSCS	Lower segment Caesarean section
LVOT	Left ventricular outflow tract
MAHA	Microangiopathic haemolytic anemia
MAP	Mean arterial pressure
MCA	Middle cerebral artery
MCH	Mean corpuscular hemoglobin

MCHC	Mean corpuscular hemoglobin concentration
MC&S	Microscopy, culture and serology
MCV	Mean corpuscular volume
MET	Metabolic equivalent
Mg	Magnesium
MI	Myocardial infarction
mmHg	Millimetres of mercury
MRCP	Magnetic resonance cholangiopancreatography
MRI	Magnetic resonance imaging
MRSA	Methicillin-resistant *Staphylococcus aureus*
Na^+	Sodium
NAP4	National Audit Project 4
NDL	Non-directed lavage
NG	Nasogastric
NICE	National Institute for Health and Care Excellence
NIHSS	National Institutes of Health Stroke Scale
NSAID	Non-steroidal anti-inflammatory drug
NSTEMI	Non-ST-segment elevation myocardial infarction
OSA	Obstructive sleep apnoea
PA	Pulmonary artery
PA	Posteroanterior
PCI	Percutaneous coronary intervention
PCR	Polymerase chain reaction
PCV	Packed cell volume
PE	Pulmonary embolism
PEEP	Positive end-expiratory pressure
PMN	Polymorphonuclear cells
PRBC	Packed red blood cells
PT	Prothrombin time
PVL	Panton-Valentine leukocidin
RAP	Right atrial pressure
RASS	Richmond Agitation Sedation Scale
RBBB	Right bundle branch block
RBC	Red blood cell
RCC	Red cell count
RCT	Randomised controlled trial
RDW	Red cell distribution width
ROTEM®	Rotational thromboelastometry

RRT	Renal replacement therapy
RSI	Rapid sequence induction
r-tPA	Recombinant tissue plasminogen activator
SAH	Subarachnoid haemorrhage
SAN	Sinoatrial node
SaO_2	Arterial oxygen saturation
SBP	Spontaneous bacterial peritonitis
$ScvO_2$	Central venous oxygen saturation
SIADH	Syndrome of inappropriate antidiuretic hormone secretion
SIRS	Systemic inflammatory response syndrome
SLE	Systemic lupus erythematosus
SR	Sinus rhythm
SSC	Surviving Sepsis Campaign
STEMI	ST-segment elevation myocardial infarction
SV	Stroke volume
SVC	Superior vena cava
SVR	Systemic vascular resistance
SVRI	Systemic vascular resistance index
SVV	Stroke volume variation
TBI	Traumatic brain injury
TBSA	Total body surface area
TEG®	Thromboelastography
TEN	Toxic epidermal necrolysis
TLS	Tumour lysis syndrome
TOE	Transoesophageal echocardiogram
TRALI	Transfusion-related acute lung injury
TT	Thrombin time
TTE	Transthoracic echocardiography
TTP	Thrombotic thrombocytopaenic purpura
U&Es	Urea and electrolytes
US	Ultrasound
VATS	Video-assisted thoracoscopic surgery
VC	Vital capacity
VHF	Viral haemorrhagic fever
WCC	White cell count

Interpreting a standard electrocardiogram (ECG)

Top Tip

Paper speed	25mm/sec
Standard voltage	10mm/mV
Each small square	0.04 seconds
Five small squares	0.2 seconds
Twenty-five small squares	1 second

Waves and intervals:

P-wave duration	0.06-0.12 seconds
	1-3 small squares
PR interval	0.12-0.2 seconds
	3-5 small squares
QRS complex duration	0.06-0.10 seconds
	1-3 small squares
QT interval	0.36-0.44 seconds

Corrected QT (QT_C) = Bazett's formula =

QT interval / $\sqrt{}$ (RR interval)

RR interval = 60/HR   0.44 seconds

A suggested structure for rapid presentation of an ECG in the OSCE scenario is presented below. Try and present all your ECGs in a set systematic manner in the lead-up to the exam, as this will allow simple marks not to be missed in the heat of your battle!

- Rate — 60 beats per minute.
- Rhythm — sinus rythm.
- Axis — left axis (-1100).
- P-wave morphology and P-R interval — normal morphology, prolonged PR.
- QRS complex — broad.
- ST segments — ST depression seen in V2, V3 (but note you cannot comment on this with bundle branch block).
- T-wave morphology — T-wave inversion V1.
- QT interval — normal.
- Is there bundle branch block? — right bundle branch block (RBBB).
- Other special notes — Q-waves in II, III aVF.

Acknowledgements

We gratefully acknowledge the following sources:

Chapter 1
Figure 1.4. Emergency tracheostomy management. © John Wiley and Sons, 2012.
McGrath BA, Bates L, Atkinson D, Moore JA. Multidisciplinary guidelines for the management of tracheostomy and laryngectomy airway emergencies. *Anaesthesia* 2012; 67(9): 1025-41.
UK National Tracheostomy Safety Project; www.tracheostomy.org.uk.

Figure 1.5. Emergency laryngectomy management. © John Wiley and Sons, 2012.
McGrath BA, Bates L, Atkinson D, Moore JA. Multidisciplinary guidelines for the management of tracheostomy and laryngectomy airway emergencies. *Anaesthesia* 2012; 67(9): 1025-41.
UK National Tracheostomy Safety Project; www.tracheostomy.org.uk.

Figure 1.6. © Dr Jeremy Jones.
Radiopaedia.org.

Figure 1.12. Algorithm for the management of CAP. © British Thoracic Society, 2009.
https://www.brit-thoracic.org.uk/guidelines-and-quality-standards/community-acquired-pneumonia-in-adults-guideline.

Chapter 2
Figure 2.12. © iStock.com/stockdevil.
http://www.istockphoto.com.

Chapter 3

Figure 3.2. Dr. Kenneth Greer. Visuals Unlimited. © Getty Images. http://www.gettyimages.co.uk.

Figure 3.4. British Thoracic Society Pleural Disease Guideline. © British Thoracic Society, 2010.
https://www.brit-thoracic.org.uk/document-library/clinical-information/pleural-disease/pleural-disease-guidelines-2010/pleural-disease-guideline-quick-reference-guide.

Chapter 4

Figure 4.3. http://www.lifeinthefastlane.com.

Figure 4.6. © C.R. Bard Inc., 2015.

Dedication

To the many teachers who took the time to teach and guide us — thank you very much. We hope that we too can contribute to this crucial continuation in medical education and training.

To our beautiful and beloved families, this book is testament to their tireless support, patience and love. We dedicate this book to you.

Jeyasankar and Daniel

Chapter 1

Acute respiratory distress syndrome (ARDS)

You are the intensive care medicine doctor on-call when you are asked to help with a patient that the nurse is finding 'difficult' to ventilate. The patient is a 45-year-old man admitted with pancreatitis 3 days ago. He was intubated on admission and his oxygen requirements have been increasing over the last 24 hours.

1) You are shown the following arterial blood gas (ABG) (● Table 1.1). Comment on the blood gas.

2 marks
(1 mark for each correct stem)

Table 1.1. Arterial blood gas results.

FiO$_2$	1.0
pH	7.35
PaO$_2$	7.4kPa
PaCO$_2$	8.9kPa
HCO$_3^-$	19mmol/L
Lacate	3.4mmol/L
BE	-10mmol/L

There is evidence of:

- Hypoxia and hypercarbia.
- A mixed respiratory and metabolic acidosis.

2) What investigations would you order?   2 marks

(0.5 mark for each correct stem, with a maximum of 2 marks)

- Chest X-ray
- Echocardiogram.
- Full blood count (FBC), urea and electrolytes (U&Es), liver function tests (LFTs), B-natriuretic peptide (BNP).
- C-reactive protein (CRP).
- Microbiological samples, e.g. sputum/broncho-alveolar lavage (BAL)/non-directed lavage (NDL).

3) You are shown the following chest X-ray (CXR) (● Figure 1.1). Comment on this CXR.   2 marks

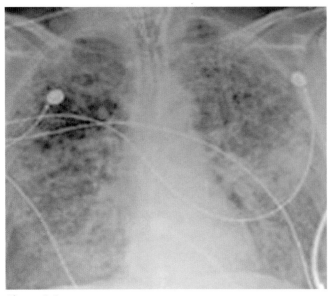

Figure 1.1.

There are the following salient features:

- An endotracheal tube *in situ*.
- Bilateral pulmonary infiltrates of a 'ground-glass' appearance.

4) What are the differential diagnoses?

4 marks

(1 mark for each correct stem, with a maximum of 4 marks)

- Acute respiratory distress syndrome (ARDS) (secondary to the pancreatitis).
- Autoimmune lung disease, e.g. Goodpasture's syndrome.
- Infection (bacterial, viral or fungal).
- Transfusion-related acute lung injury (TRALI).
- Pulmonary fibrosis.
- Pulmonary haemorrhage.
- Interstitial oedema.
- *Pneumocystis jirovecii* pneumonia (PJP) infection.
- Cardiac failure or valvular heart disease.
- Toxic shock syndrome.

5) What other key imaging would you request?

1 mark

- CT of the chest.

6)   Comment on this scan (● Figure 1.2).   2 marks

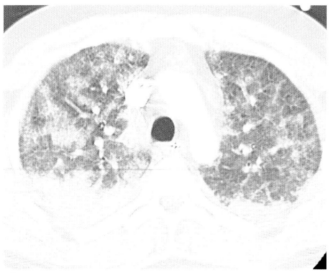

Figure 1.2.

- There is ground-glass shadowing with bilateral pleural effusions.
- This is consistent with ARDS.

7)   How would you ventilate this patient?

4 marks
(1 mark for each correct stem)

The ARDSnet ventilatory strategies should be implemented [1]:

- Tidal volumes 6-8ml/kg ideal body weight.
- Plateau pressure <30cmH$_2$O.
- Positive end-expiratory pressure (PEEP) titrated to FiO$_2$.
- Permissive hypercapnia.

8) The patient continues to deteriorate. What other strategies with proven positive evidence are there to improve severe ARDS and refractory hypoxia?

3 marks
(1 mark for each correct stem)

The following strategies have supporting current evidence in improving the outcome in severe ARDS cases:

- Prone positioning of the patient. There was an improved mortality in severe ARDS as recently shown in the PROSEVA trial [2].
- Muscle relaxation or paralysis. The ACURASYS trial found an improvement in mortality with the early implementation of a cisatracurium infusion in cases of severe ARDS [3].
- Extracorporeal membrane oxygenation (ECMO). The CESAR trial demonstrated an improvement in oxygenation in patients with severe ARDS [4].

Top Tip

The OSCE exam will often ask for a 'list' of answers; for example, please list some causes, differential diagnoses, specific investigations, etc. It is important to recognise that time is a precious commodity and that the list needs to be produced in a succinct and swift manner. In order to help with this it is well worth having a system to organise your answer and in the days approaching the exam to practice these systems in producing answers. For example, in the question above on listing some differential diagnoses for the CXR, a simple system could be utilising the classic surgical sieve, 'VITAMIN C', or using the body systems to list potential causes. So in this example the causes for this CXR could be organised as such:

- **V**ascular — pulmonary infarction or congestive cardiac failure.
- **I**atrogenic — fluid overload from excessive blood product or intravenous fluid administration.
- **T**raumatic — pulmonary contusions.
- **A**utoimmune — Goodpasture's syndrome, severe sarcoid disease or systemic lupus erythematosus (SLE).
- **M**etabolic.
- **I**nfective or inflammatory:
  - infective causes subclassified as bacterial, viral, protozoal or fungal. In this case many organisms could have precipitated such a chest radiograph;
  - inflammatory causes — ARDS.
- **N**eoplastic.
- **C**ongenital.

References

1. http://www.ardsnet.org/system/files/Ventilator%20Protocol%20 Card.pdf.

2. Guerin C, Reignier J, Richard JC, *et al*. Prone positioning in severe acute respiratory distress syndrome. *N Engl J Med* 2013; 368: 2159-68.

3. Papazian L, Forel JM, Gacouin A, *et al*. Neuromuscular blockers in early acute respiratory distress syndrome. *N Engl J Med* 2010; 363: 1107-16.

4. Peek GJ, Clemens F, Elbourne D, *et al*. CESAR: Conventional Ventilatory Support vs. Extracorporeal Membrane Oxygenation for Severe Adult Respiratory Failure. *BMC Health Services Research* 2006; 6: 163.

Cardiac output monitoring

This station will explore different aspects of cardiac output monitors.

1) What form of cardiac monitoring does this picture represent (● Figure 1.3)?   1 mark

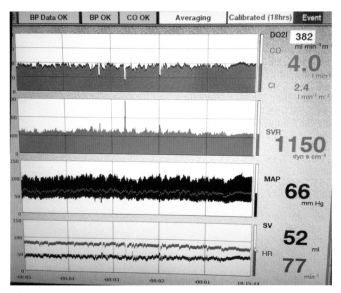

Figure 1.3.

This is a screen-shot of the information derived from a cardiac output monitor:

● Pulse contour wave analysis.
● Specifically lithium dilution cardiac output monitoring (LIDCO).

2)   Below are some values from a cardiac output   6 marks
     monitor (● Table 1.2). Please summarise the
     information and explain what this indicates.

Table 1.2. Summary from a cardiac output monitor.	
HR	50 bpm
MAP	52mmHg
CO	2.5L/min
CI	1.3L/min/m^2
SV	49ml
DO$_2$I	171ml/min/m^2
SVRI	2850dyne/sec/cm^5/m^2
Venous saturation	80%

Key points in summary:

● The heart rate is low.
● The patient is hypotensive in spite of a high systemic vascular resistance (SVR).
● The cardiac output (CO) indices are all low with a low oxygen delivery.

Key points in the explanation:

● The CO is low as a result of a low heart rate or filling.
● The raised SVR will contribute to a raised afterload increasing the work of the heart and potentially decreasing the CO.

- The CO is low for this body's surface area as the oxygen delivery is compromised as well.

3) **What are the principles of pulse waveform contour analysis?**   1 mark

- An arterial waveform trace can be analysed within the context of the patient's heart rate, weight and height.
- Stroke volume (SV) is proportional to the area under the curve up to the dicrotic notch.

4) **Which values are measured and which are calculated?**

2 marks
(1 mark for each correct stem, with a maximum of 2 marks)

- Information that can be directly measured include the heart rate (HR), blood pressure (BP) and mean arterial pressure (MAP).
- Information that can be calculated include the SV and CO.
- Information that can be derived include the cardiac index (CI), oxygen delivery index (DO_2I) and systemic vascular resistance index (SVRI).

5) **What are some of the management options or strategies that could be employed for this patient to improve cardiac output?**

3 marks
(1 mark for each correct stem)

- Increase the heart rate.
- Improve intravascular filling and, hence, venous return which may improve the MAP.
- Improve the afterload by decreasing the SVR.

6) This patient has an SVV of 18%. What is the SVV and what management strategy could be undertaken based on this information?

3 marks
(0.5 mark for each correct stem)

- Stroke volume variation (SVV) is a marker of fluid responsiveness.
- It is the percentage change in SV that occurs during the ventilator cycle.
- The normal SVV is 5-10%.
- Fluid challenges of approximately 150-250ml of IV fluid could be given which should improve cardiac preload. This may be transient.
- If an improvement in SVV and SV are seen then a further fluid challenge should be undertaken.
- Fluid challenges should continue to be given until the SVV no longer responds.

7) List some other cardiac output monitors.

2 marks
(0.5 mark for each correct stem, with a maximum of 2 marks)

- Oesophageal Doppler.
- Other pulse contour analysis tools — LIDCO, PICCO.
- Pulmonary artery catheter.
- Transthoracic echocardiogram.
- Transoesophageal echocardiogram.

8) With regard to oesophageal Doppler, what unique values can be derived from it and what do they represent?

2 marks

- Peak velocity — an indication of ventricular contractility.
- Flow time corrected — duration of flow during systole. This is an indicator of preload or afterload.

References

1. Chamos C, Vele L, Hamilton M, Cecconi M. Less invasive methods of advanced hemodynamic monitoring: principles, devices, and their role in the perioperative hemodynamic optimization. *Perioper Med* 2013; 2: 19.

Tracheostomy emergency

You are the doctor on the intensive care unit (ICU). You are asked to see a patient whom the nursing staff are having difficulty ventilating. He is a 75-year-old gentleman who has been on the ICU for some time and is currently being weaned from the ventilator. He had a tracheostomy placed to facilitate his wean 2 weeks ago.

An examiner will play the part of the nurse looking after the patient and you will be presented with a manikin, with a tracheostomy tube in place attached to a ventilator circuit.

This OSCE and mark sheet follows the National Tracheostomy Safety Project guidelines, of which the key algorithms are presented below (● Figures 1.4 and 1.5).

The OSCE will follow in the order listed below, with marks awarded for the candidate demonstrating the following key manoeuvres OR equally declaring that they would do so.

1) The candidate:

- Takes a brief history from the nurse whilst assessing breathing.   1 mark
- Applies high-flow oxygen to the mouth.   1 mark
- Applies a Mapleson C circuit with high-flow oxygen to the tracheostomy.   2 marks
- Asks for capnography.   1 mark
- Calls for 'expert' airway help and the difficult airway trolley.   2 marks
- Establishes that the patient is not breathing.   1 mark

- Attempts to ventilate the patient via a tracheostomy.   2 marks
- Checks if the tracheostomy tube has an inner tube   1 mark
  and removes this if present.
- Attempts to pass a suction catheter down the   1 mark
  tracheostomy tube.

2) The candidate is informed that in this scenario   1 mark
   they are unable to pass the suction catheter.
   The candidate needs to demonstrate that
   they:

- Deflate the cuff on the tracheostomy, and assess for
  signs of breathing.

3) The patient still shows no signs of breathing.
   The candidate needs to:

- Remove the tracheostomy tube and reassess, ensuring   1 mark
  that oxygen is applied to both the mouth and stoma.
- Cover the stoma with swabs and attempt bag mask   2 marks
  ventilation.
- Use appropriate airway manoeuvres and adjuncts.   1 mark

4) The candidate is informed that again in this   2 marks
   scenario they are unable to ventilate the
   patient. The candidate should then
   demonstrate that they:

- Insert a supraglottic airway and attempt to gently
  ventilate.

5) This is successful. The candidate is asked to explain their next step which is: 1 mark

- Plans for endotracheal intubation in a safe and controlled manner.

References

1.   McGrath BA, Bates L, Atkinson D, Moore JA. Multidisciplinary guidelines for the management of tracheostomy and laryngectomy airway emergencies. *Anaesthesia* 2012; 67(9): 1025-41.

The two algorithms overleaf are reproduced from McGrath BA, Bates L, Atkinson D, Moore JA. Multidisciplinary guidelines for the management of tracheostomy and laryngectomy airway emergencies. Anaesthesia 2012; 67(9): 1025-41, with permission from the Association of Anaesthetists of Great Britain & Ireland/© John Wiley and Sons, 2012.

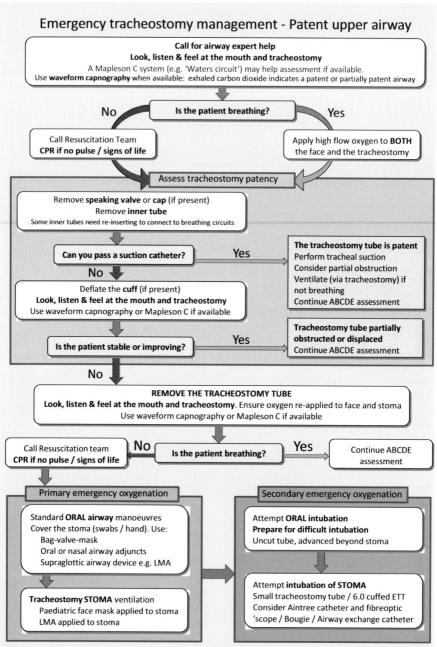

Figure 1.4. Emergency tracheostomy management.

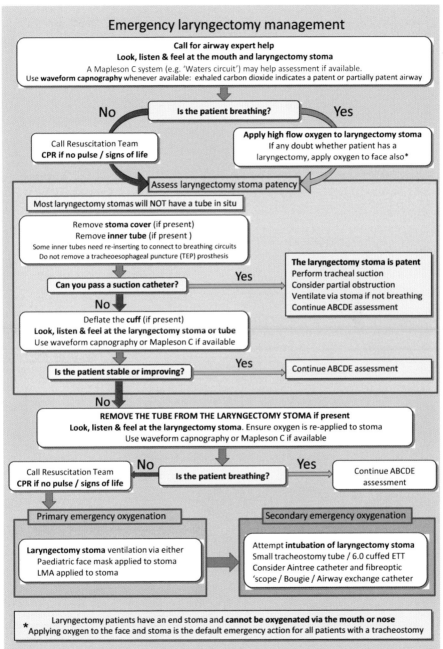

Emergency laryngectomy management

Call for airway expert help
Look, listen & feel at the mouth and laryngectomy stoma
A Mapleson C system (e.g. 'Waters circuit') may help assessment if available.
Use **waveform capnography** whenever available: exhaled carbon dioxide indicates a patent or partially patent airway

No   **Is the patient breathing?**   **Yes**

Call Resuscitation Team
CPR if no pulse / signs of life

Apply high flow oxygen to laryngectomy stoma
If any doubt whether patient has a
laryngectomy, apply oxygen to face also*

Assess laryngectomy stoma patency

Most laryngectomy stomas will NOT have a tube in situ

Remove **stoma cover** (if present)
Remove **inner tube** (if present)
Some inner tubes need re-inserting to connect to breathing circuits
Do not remove a tracheoesophageal puncture (TEP) prosthesis

Can you pass a suction catheter?   **Yes**
No

The laryngectomy stoma is patent
Perform tracheal suction
Consider partial obstruction
Ventilate via stoma if not breathing
Continue ABCDE assessment

Deflate the **cuff** (if present)
Look, listen & feel at the laryngectomy stoma or tube
Use waveform capnography or Mapleson C if available

Is the patient stable or improving?   **Yes** → Continue ABCDE assessment
No

REMOVE THE TUBE FROM THE LARYNGECTOMY STOMA if present
Look, listen & feel at the laryngectomy stoma. Ensure oxygen is re-applied to stoma
Use waveform capnography or Mapleson C if available

Call Resuscitation Team
CPR if no pulse / signs of life
No   **Is the patient breathing?**   **Yes** → Continue ABCDE
assessment

Primary emergency oxygenation

Laryngectomy stoma ventilation via either
Paediatric face mask applied to stoma
LMA applied to stoma

Secondary emergency oxygenation

Attempt **intubation of laryngectomy stoma**
Small tracheostomy tube / 6.0 cuffed ETT
Consider Aintree catheter and fibreoptic
'scope / Bougie / Airway exchange catheter

* Laryngectomy patients have an end stoma and **cannot be oxygenated via the mouth or nose**
Applying oxygen to the face and stoma is the default emergency action for all patients with a tracheostomy

National Tracheostomy Safety Project. Review date 1/4/14. Feedback & resources at **www.tracheostomy.org.uk**

Figure 1.5. Emergency laryngectomy management.

17

Corticosteroids in the ICU

A 32-year-old man is in the emergency medicine resuscitation bay requiring critical care review. The patient has a 7-week history of progressively worsening fatigue.

1) The patient has the following observations and biochemistry results (● Table 1.3). Summarise your findings.

2 marks
(0.5 mark for each correct stem)

Table 1.3. Observations and biochemistry results.

BP	89/37mmHg
HR	110 bpm
GCS	10/15 (E2 M5 V3)
Temp	35.9°C
Na^+	121mmol/L
K^+	5.4mmol/L
Cl^-	72mmol/L
HCO_3^-	16mmol/L
Urea	16.1mmol/L
Creatinine	128μmol/L

- Hypotensive, tachycardic patient with a low GCS indicating poor cerebral perfusion.
- Hyponatraemia and hyperkalaemia.
- Low bicarbonate indicative of a severe metabolic acidosis.
- Raised urea out of proportion to the creatinine, indicative of hypovolaemia or intravascular depletion.

2) The following results (● Table 1.4) are presented to you. What do they indicate?   2 marks

Table 1.4. Paired urine and plasma osmolalities.

Serum osmolality	224mosm/kg
Urine osmolality	162mosm/kg
Urine sodium	<20mmol/L

- Severe hypovolaemia.
- Hyponatraemia.

3) What is your immediate management plan?

- Acute assessment, resuscitation and management should be undertaken to follow an 'airway, breathing, circulation, disability and exposure' approach.   0.5 mark
- IV — fluid resuscitation.   1 mark
- Short synacthen or cosyntropin test.   0.5 mark
- IV corticosteroids (high dose).   1 mark

4) The following test results are obtained (● Table 1.5). What is your most likely diagnosis?   1 mark

Table 1.5. Further test results.

Random cortisol	<0.2μg/dL
250μg of cosyntropin	The cortisol level remained <0.2μg/dL
Adrenocorticotrophic hormone (ACTH)	742pg/dL (5-27pg/dL)

19

- Primary Addison's disease.

5) Classify the causes of adrenal insufficiency — inadequate basal cortisol.

5 marks

(3 marks for primary Addison's disease with two causes, 1 mark each for secondary and tertiary causes with a correct explanation)

(If the candidate does not identify the diagnosis then ask for the causes of adrenal insufficiency.)

Primary Addison's disease:

- Autoimmune adrenalitis.
- Haemorrhage.
- Malignancy — primary tumour or metastatic lesions.
- Infection — TB, meningococcal.
- Inflammatory.

Secondary:

- Insufficient ACTH production secondary to pituitary pathology.

Tertiary:

- Adrenal atrophy secondary to exogenous corticosteroid suppression.

6) List five reasons for corticosteroid use in the critical care setting.

5 marks

- Airway — croup or post-op ENT/maxillofacial surgery.

- Breathing:
  - anaphylaxis;
  - pneumonia;
  - chronic obstructive pulmonary disease (COPD);
  - *Pneumocystis jirovecii*.

- Circulation:
  - vasopressor refractive shock, for example, in septic shock.

- Endocrine:
  - Addison's disease;
  - hypercalcaemia;
  - Addisonian crisis — in patients who have been on long-term steroid use.

- Nervous system:
  - myasthenic crisis;
  - myxoedema coma;
  - brain tumour swelling;
  - bacterial meningitis.

- Organ donation — post brainstem death testing.
- Malignancy.

7) What is the role of the short synacthen test and steroids in severe sepsis or septic shock?

- The test is not recommended as routine practice in severe sepsis or septic shock (Surviving Sepsis Guidelines, 2012 [1]).

0.5 mark

- Due to a variation in the free cortisol fraction the adrenal function cannot be accurately assessed in sepsis. 0.5 mark

- The Surviving Sepsis Guidelines have made a recommendation that corticosteroids (CCS) can be used in vasopressor refractive shock. 1 mark

References

1.   Surviving Sepsis Guidelines. http://www.sccm.org/Documents/SSC-Guidelines.pdf.

Blood product transfusion

You are the doctor on the ICU and have been called to the emergency department as part of the trauma team where a lady has been admitted following a road traffic accident. She is hypotensive and is about to undergo a 4-unit blood transfusion prior to going to theatre for urgent surgery.

You are asked by the nurse if you would check the blood before the transfusion is commenced.

In this scenario the examiner will act as the nurse, and there will be a manikin arm, with a patient identification (ID) band around the wrist. There will also be four model blood bags with their respective tags, a transfusion slip and a drug chart.

The OSCE will follow in the order listed below, with marks awarded for the candidate demonstrating the following key manoeuvres OR equally declaring that they would do so.

1) The candidate declares that they would: 4 marks

- Attempt to gain consent for transfusion and states if consent cannot be gained in, for example, an intubated and sedated patient, that the transfusion will be in the patient's 'best interest'.
- Attempt to positively identify the patient (i.e. asks the patient their name and date of birth).

- Ask another member of staff to check the patient's details against the name band and patient's drug chart.
- Ensure the blood is prescribed.

Remember the minimum data set is first name, surname, date of birth, hospital identification number or code.

2) The candidate demonstrates or declares that they would: 6 marks

- Visually check the blood bags for any damage.
- Check expiry dates.
- Check that the details match on the patient's ID band, blood bag tag and transfusion slip, and that they all match correctly.
- Check that the blood group and donation number on the bag and tag are identical.
- Check these against the transfusion slip.
- Check that this is done for each of the units to be transfused.

3) How long can blood remain out of the fridge before it needs to be transfused?   1 mark

- Less than 4 hours.

4) The patient's blood group is A positive. Which   2 marks
    blood groups can this patient be transfused?

- O positive, O negative.
- A positive, A negative.

5) She is brought to the ICU following her surgery   2 marks
    and 2 hours later becomes difficult to   (1 mark for
    ventilate. A chest X-ray is ordered (● Figure   each correct
    1.6). What are your differential diagnoses?   stem, with a
    maximum of 2
    marks)

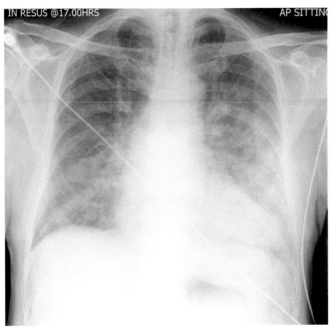

Figure 1.6.

- Transfusion-related acute lung injury (TRALI).
- Acute fluid overload.
- Acute respiratory distress syndrome (ARDS).

6) **Why has this complication become less common?** 1 mark

- Blood products are leukodepleted as standard practice.

7) **What are the other potential complications when transfusing a significant amount of blood?** 4 marks
(1 mark for each correct stem, with a maximum of 4 marks)

- Hypothermia.
- Coagulopathy.
- Congestive cardiac failure (CCF).
- Thrombocytopaenia.
- Hypocalcaemia.
- Hyperkalaemia.

References

1. NHS Professional Clinical Guideline (CG4).
    http://www.nhsprofessionals.nhs.uk/download/comms/cg4%20-%20blood%20transfusion%20guidelines.pdf.

Diabetic ketoacidosis

A 21-year-old newly diagnosed diabetic is admitted to the emergency department following a night out. The patient was believed to have had an evening of excess alcohol. The patient is drowsy and agitated.

1) Review and present the findings of this ABG (● Table 1.6).

1 mark
(0.5 mark for each correct stem)

Table 1.6. Arterial blood gas results.

pH	6.89
PaO_2	11.0kPa
$PaCO_2$	3.2kPa
HCO_3^-	12mmol/L
BE	-12.1mmol/L
Blood glucose	27mmol/L

- There is a metabolic acidosis with failed respiratory compensation.
- Raised blood sugar.

2) What is the most likely diagnosis?

1 mark
(0.5 mark for each correct stem)

- A diabetic emergency:
  - likely to be diabetic ketoacidosis (DKA);
  - hyperglycaemic, hyperosmolar state (HHS).

3) What further tests are required to confirm the diagnosis? 0.5 mark

● Urine or blood ketones.

4) A ketonaemia is discovered at 6.2mmol/L. What are the principles in the management of DKA?

4 marks
(1 mark for each correct stem, with a maximum of 4 marks)

● The primary goal and priority is ketone clearance.
● Fluid resuscitation.
● Insulin replacement.
● Controlled glucose reduction.
● Treatment of a precipitant cause — for example, antibiotics for concurrent infection.

5) What guidelines are you aware of which have directed the management of DKA?

1 mark
(a mark will be given for any relevant national guideline)

● The Joint British Diabetes Societies (JBDS) guidelines for the management of DKA.

6) According to the guidelines by the BDS what are the rates of change that are targeted for ketones, bicarbonate and glucose?

3 marks

● Rate of fall for ketones — 0.5mmol/L/hr.
● Rate of rise in HCO_3^- — 3mmol/L/hr.
● Rate of fall for glucose — 3mmol/L.

7) What type of fluid would you use and what regime would you follow?

- Normal saline.   0.5 mark
- If the patient is hypotensive, with a systolic pressure   0.5 mark
  less than 90mmHg, give 0.5L of fluid in 15 mins.
- Otherwise: 0.5 mark
  - 0.5L in 15mins;
  - 1L in 1 hour;
  - 1L in 2 hours;
  - 1L in 4 hours;
  - 1L in 4 hours;
  - 1L in 6 hours.
- If K^+ is less than 5mmol/L, then supplement the   0.5 mark
  normal saline with potassium chloride.
- When glucose is <14mmol/L, add in 10% dextrose   1 mark
  at 125ml/hr.

8) What patient group would this fluid resuscitation regime not be used and why?

2 marks
(0.5 mark for each correct stem)

- Young 18-25 — cerebral oedema.
- Elderly — fluid overload.
- Hepatic and renal failure — fluid overload.
- Pregnancy — cerebral oedema.

9) What rate of insulin administration would you institute and until what point would you continue insulin?

2 marks

- 0.1 units/kg/hr.
- Continue until the ketone level is <0.3mmol/L.

10) **What are the main differences in fluid and insulin regimes in a hyperglycaemic hyperosmolar state (HHS) and why?**

2 marks (1 mark for each correct stem, with a maximum of 2 marks)

- In a HHS, there is severe dehydration, but due to the high risk of cerebral oedema the initial fluid replacement is slower compared to DKA; approximately 6L in a 24-hour period.
- Slower insulin regime of 0.05 units/kg/hr but only after fluid resuscitation.
- Slow correction of hypernatraemia due to the risk of central pontine myolinolysis.

11) **What collection of events are both HHS and DKA patients at high risk of?**

0.5 mark

- Thromboembolic events including deep venous thrombosis (DVT), pulmonary embolism (PE), cerebrovascular accident (CVA) or myocardial infarction (MI).

References

1.   http://www.diabetes.org.uk/Documents/About%20Us/What%20we%20say/Management-of-DKA-241013.pdf.

Professionalism — critical incident reporting

You are the ICU doctor and have been asked to talk to the junior doctor who was on-call at night over the weekend.

The patient, who was admitted for an upper gastrointestinal (GI) bleed, was transfused during resuscitation on the unit. In total he received 20 units of packed red cells; however, when the blood bank checked the transfusion slips, two of the slips had another patient's details on them. It would appear that he was transfused with another patient's cross-matched blood. The patient eventually went for endoscopy where a bleeding point was identified and he was stabilised and is currently still on the ICU.

This station will have an actor playing the part of the junior colleague.

1) Please discuss the case with the junior doctor and outline the next steps with regard to this incident.

The candidate:

- Provides an appropriate introduction, including their name, grade and role.   1 mark
- Ascertains the junior doctor's name, and explains the purpose of the discussion.   1 mark
- Checks that the junior doctor is happy to continue and does not want anyone else present.   1 mark
- Allows the junior doctor to tell his/her side of the story without interruption.   1 mark

- Outlines the incident to the junior doctor and explains that this is a 'critical incident'.   1 mark
- Explains that this will need to be investigated, and an incident form filled out.   1 mark
- Explains that the investigation is not to apportion blame but to try to prevent such events from happening again.   2 marks
- Outlines the mechanism for critical incident reporting.   2 marks
- States that this particular error is a 'never event' and explains what this means.   3 marks
- When asked not to report it by the junior doctor, informs him/her that it will be reported.   1 mark
- Offers support mechanisms for the junior doctor, e.g. educational supervisor, college tutor, Medical Defence Union.   2 marks
- Informs the junior doctor that this will need to be recorded on his/her revalidation documentation.   1 mark
- Is non-judgemental, and uses clear and appropriate language.   2 marks
- Closes the discussion appropriately.   1 mark

References

1. http://www.npsa.nhs.uk/nrls/reporting/what-is-a-patient-safety-incident.
2. Mahajan RP. Critical incident reporting and learning. *Br J Anaesth* 2010; 105(1): 69-75.

Equipment

1)   What is this piece of equipment (● Figure 1.7)?   1 mark

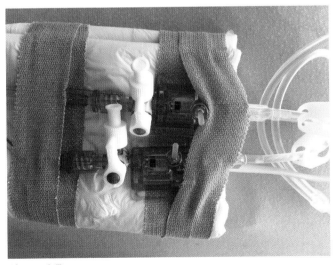

Figure 1.7.

- This is a pressure transducer.

2) **What does this piece of equipment measure?** 2 marks

(0.5 mark for
each correct
stem)

- This is used as part of a set of equipment to measure a variety of intravascular or intracompartmental pressures. It is commonly used to measure:
  - invasive blood pressures;
  - central venous pressures;
  - intra-abdominal pressures;
  - intracranial pressures.

3) **What is a transducer?** 1 mark

- A transducer converts energy from one form into another form of energy.

4) **In the context of an invasive arterial blood pressure (IABP) monitoring system, how does a transducer work?** 1 mark

- In an IABP monitoring system, arterial pressure changes are converted into electrical signals by the transducer which are then measured, analysed, processed and displayed.

5) **You are presented with this picture below (● Figure 1.8). The pressure transducer is part of a system. What are the basic components of this system when measuring invasive arterial blood pressure (IABP)?** 5 marks

(1 mark for
each correct
stem)

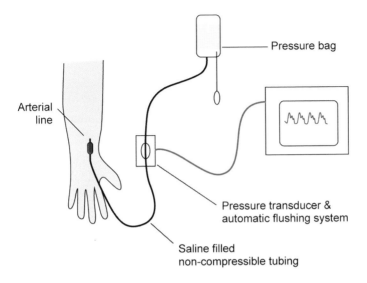

Figure 1.8.

- A catheter or arterial line placed in the artery.
- An incompressible rigid or stiff-walled, fluid-filled piece of tubing.
- A pressure transducer.
- Bag of fluid in a pressure bag with fluid (usually 0.9% saline or heparinised 0.9% saline) pressurised to 300mmHg to maintain the column of fluid in the system, and also deliver a flushing capability.
- Electronic receiving device which computes the information and presents the information as a number and waveform.

6) **What is the mechanism behind the system in measuring IABP?**

5 marks
(1 mark for each correct stem)

- The catheter is in direct continuation with the column of fluid held under pressure in the rigid tubing.
- Intra-arterial pulsations are carried through this column to the pressure transducer where a sensitive diaphragm attached to a strain gauge is present.
- This forms part of a Wheatstone bridge set of resistors.
- Changes in the pulsations deform the diaphragm with changes in strain gauge resistance sensed by the electronic receiving device.
- Fourier analysis is used to construct a wave form and calculate the blood pressure details.

7) **What is damping in the context of the IABP system?**

2 marks
(1 mark for each correct stem)

- The IABP measuring system relies on the carriage of oscillations from the artery to the transducer.
- Damping reduces the amplitude of these oscillations; for example, due to air bubbles or blood clots in the column of fluid, kinks in the tubing or compliant, long tubing.

8) **What are the characteristics of an arterial catheter which prevents overdamping?**

1 mark

- A short, wide and non-compliant piece of tubing.

9) What is optimal damping (● Figure 1.9 and ● Table 1.7)?

2 marks
(1 mark for each correct stem)

- The coefficient of damping is 0.7.
- This is a compromise between overdamping, underdamping, speed and accuracy.

Top Tip

Fast flush test. This can easily feature as a potential part of this question. The flush feature on the highly pressurised bag causes an undershoot and overshoot of waves, before finally settling around the natural frequency of the system. The flush test can be used to determine the damping coefficient. The identification and familiarity of the waveforms below could be asked.

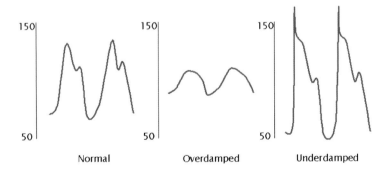

Figure 1.9. The effects of damping on the arterial wave form.

Table 1.7. Arterial trace damping and their relative coefficients.

Critical damping	Damping coefficient of 1.0
Over-damping	Damping coefficient >1.0
Under-damping	Damping coefficient <1.0
Optimal-damping	Damping coefficient 0.7

References

1. Ward M, Langton JA. Blood pressure measurement. *Cont Educ Anaesth Crit Care Pain* 2007; 7(4): 122-6.

Community-acquired pneumonia

A 78-year-old man presents to the emergency department with a 3-day history of shortness of breath, fever and a productive cough. He is currently in the resuscitation section of the emergency department breathing high-flow oxygen via a non-rebreathe mask. His respiratory rate is 32 breaths per minute, heart rate is 120 bpm and blood pressure is 101/62mmHg. His temperature is 39.4°C.

1) You are asked to review the patient. On arrival in the emergency department you are presented with the following blood results (Table 1.8). Please comment on the results.

3 marks

Table 1.8. Blood test results.	
Hb	101g/L
WCC	21.1 x 10^9/L
Platelets	347 x 10^9/L
MCV	101fL
PCV	0.46L/L
RBC	5.4 x 10^{12}/L
MCH	29pg
MCHC	324g/L
RDW	12.3%
Neutrophils	17.6 x 10^9/L
Lymphocytes	1.8 x 10^9/L
Monocytes	0.8 x 10^9/L
Eosinophils	0.6 x 10^9/L

Continued overleaf

Table 1.8. Blood test results *continued*.	
Na$^+$	143mmol/L
K$^+$	4.2mmol/L
Urea	11.3mmol/L
Creatinine	145μmol/L
CRP	129mg/L
pH	7.45
PO$_2$	8.5kPa
PCO$_2$	4.3kPa
HCO$_3^-$	21.2mmol/L
Cl$^-$	97mmol/L
Lactate	2.5mmol/L
BE	-4.5mmol/L

There is:

- A high white cell count (neutrophilia).
- An increased CRP.
- Evidence of an acute kidney injury (AKI).
- A large A/a gradient.
- A metabolic acidosis with respiratory compensation.

2) **What other tests/investigations would you like to request?**

2 marks
(0.5 mark for each correct stem, with a maximum of 2 marks)

- Chest X-ray.
- Electrocardiogram.
- Troponin.
- Blood culture.

- Urine dipstick to include *Legionella* and Pneumococcal urinary antigens.
- Sputum culture.

3) A chest X-Ray is performed (Figure 1.10). 1 mark
Please describe the abnormality.

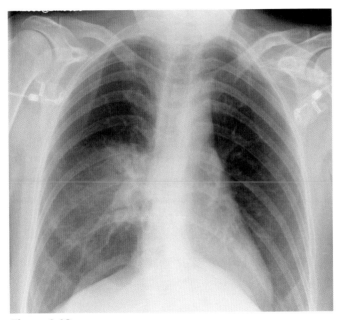

Figure 1.10.

- There is a right middle lobe pneumonia.

4) How would you risk stratify this patient? 2 marks
(for naming of the scoring system and its individual components)

The CURB65 scoring system can be used:

- Confusion (new onset) — Abbreviated Mental Test Score (AMTS) <8.
- Urea >7mmol/L.
- Respiratory rate >30 breaths per minute.
- Blood pressure — systolic <90mmHg or diastolic <60mmHg.
- Age >65.

The total number of points is then totalled with the following inference for further care:

2 marks
(for correctly listing the total criteria and inference)

- 0-1 — treatment in the community.
- 2-3 — hospital admission.
- 4-5 — critical care admission.

Top Tip

Commonly utilised scoring systems in intensive care medicine are often explored in the ICM exams. Knowledge of the scoring system with its application and implication on the patient in the OSCE scenario is an important part of the exam. In this case one could also mention the Pneumonia Severity Index. Although this is more accurate in predicting mortality it is a more complicated score to calculate.

5) **Which causative organisms are most likely in this patient?**

3 marks
(1 mark for each correct stem, with a maximum of 3 marks)

- *Streptococcus pneumoniae.*
- *Haemophilus influenzae.*

- Atypical organisms (e.g. *Mycoplasma pneumoniae*, *Legionella pneumophila*).
- Viral (e.g. influenza, parainfluenza).

6) How would you treat this patient?

3 marks
(1 mark for each correct stem, with a maximum of 3 marks)

The following measures should be implemented:

- Acute assessment, resuscitation and management should be undertaken to follow an 'airway, breathing, circulation, disability and exposure' approach.
- Management to follow care bundles as listed by the Surviving Sepsis Campaign.
- Early antibiotics, including cover for atypical organisms.
- An antimicrobial regime which has coverage for both typical and atypical organisms causing community-acquired pneumonia, e.g. benzyl penicillin and clarithromycin.

7) How would your antibiotic choice change if this patient had developed pneumonia in hospital?

2 marks
(0.5 mark for each correct stem, with a maximum of 2 marks)

- It would be necessary to cover for nosocomial infections.
- Most hospital-acquired infections are Gram-negative organisms, so antimicrobial cover would be required to cover these.
- Methicillin-resistant *Staphylococcus aureus* (MRSA) coverage will be required if the patient is MRSA screen-positive or fails to improve with initial therapy.
- An alternative antimicrobial regime, e.g. piperacillin-tazobactam.

8) The patient has the following chest X-ray on day 5 of his hospital stay (● Figure 1.11). Please comment on this chest X-ray.   1 mark

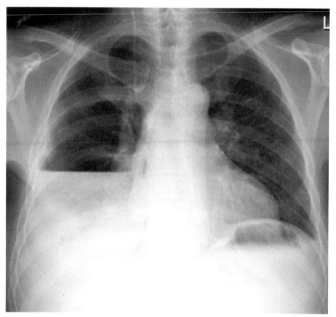

Figure 1.11.

- There is a right-sided empyema.

9) How would you treat this pathology?   1 mark

- As antibiotics have appeared to fail, the patient would need an intercostal drain.

The flow chart below is from the BTS guidance for CAP (● Figure 1.12).

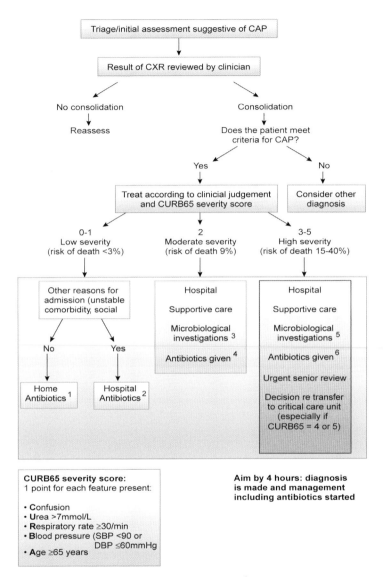

Figure 1.12. Algorithm for the management of CAP.

1 For example, amoxicillin 500mg tds orally OR clarithromycin 500mg bd orally.

2 For example, amoxicillin 500mg tds orally or intravenously OR clarithromycin 500mg bd orally.

Continued overleaf

3 Investigations for moderate risk include blood cultures, sputum microscopy, culture and sensitivities (MC&S), pneumococcal urine antigen test, pleural fluid if present for MC&S and pneumococcal antigen, PCR or serological investigations, urine *Legionella* antigen, sputum for *Legionella* culture and direct immunofluorescence (if available).

4 For example, amoxicillin 500mg-1g tds orally or intravenously AND clarithromycin 500mg bd orally or intravenously.

5 Investigations same as for moderate risk, but further inclusive of sputum for PCR for *Mycoplasma pneumoniae*, *Chlamydia spp.*, influenza A and B, parainfluenza 1-3, adenovirus, respiratory syncytial virus and *Pneumocystis jirovecii* (if at risk).

6 For example, co-amoxiclav 1.2g tds intravenously AND clarithromycin 500mg bd intravenously. If *Legionella* suspected, then add in levofloxacin.

For the full guidelines please refer to the "2015 — Annotated BTS Guideline for the management of CAP in adults (2009) — Summary of recommendations".
https://www.brit-thoracic.org.uk/guidelines-and-quality-standards/community-acquired-pneumonia-in-adults-guideline/. © British Thoracic Society, 2009.

References

1. 2015 - Annotated BTS Guideline for the management of CAP in adults (2009) - Summary of recommendations. https://www.brit-thoracic.org.uk/guidelines-and-quality-standards/community-acquired-pneumonia-in-adults-guideline/.

Guillain-Barré syndrome and plasmapheresis

A 52-year-old lady has presented to hospital with progressively worsening weakness in her legs and pins and needles in her hands. She had been recovering from an upper respiratory tract infection approximately 2 weeks prior to the development of these symptoms. She had no other medical or surgical history of note. During the course of her 24-hour stay the weakness had progressed and ventilation was starting to become a problem. You are called to review the patient.

1) What is the most likely diagnosis?   1 mark

- Guillain-Barré syndrome (acute inflammatory demyelinating polyneuropathy).

2) What is Guillain-Barré syndrome?   3 marks

- An acute, immune-mediated, inflammatory, polyneuropathy.
- It is characterised by progressive symmetrical weakness, and sensory and autonomic instability.

3) What investigations would you carry out for a patient with suspected Guillain-Barré syndrome?

- Bloods — FBC, U&Es, LFTs, a vasculitic screen, erythrocyte sedimentation rate (ESR).   0.5 mark
- Antibody tests.   0.5 mark

- Radiological — CXR, MRI.   0.5 mark
- Protein electrophoresis.   0.5 mark
- Cerebrospinal fluid (CSF) — looking for raised protein   1 mark
  levels with a normal white cell count (1 mark with
  justification), and oligoclonal bands indicative of
  multiple sclerosis (0.5 mark given if this is the only
  justification for CSF).
- Nerve conduction studies — depicting disturbance in   1 mark
  the speed of nerve conduction in keeping with an
  inflammatory demyelinating polyneuropathy.

4) What other tests would you do in relation to a   2 marks
   preceding prodromal infection?

- Blood microscopy, culture and serology (MC&S).
- CSF MC&S.
- Stool MC&S — including for *Campylobacter*.
- Throat swabs — for *Streptococci*.
- Viral serology — *Varicella zoster* and *Herpes simplex*.

5) In addition to 'ABCDE' what are the specific   3 marks
   management options in Guillain-Barré
   syndrome?

- High-dose steroids.
- Intravenous immunoglobulins.
- Plasmapheresis.

6) What is plasmapheresis?   2 marks

- It is the extracorporeal purification of blood where
  certain constituents of plasma are removed by either

membrane filtration or centrifugation. A replacement fluid is then added such as albumin, fresh frozen plasma (FFP) or cryoprecipitate and returned to the body with the patient's blood.

7) List four clinical conditions or circumstances where plasmapheresis can be of therapeutic value.

2 marks

- Guillain-Barré syndrome.
- Myasthenia gravis.
- Thrombotic thrombocytopaenic purpura.
- Systemic lupus erythematosus (SLE).
- Multiple myeloma.
- Plasma protein bound intoxication too large for renal replacement therapy, for example, digoxin toxicity.

8) List some complications of plasmapheresis.

3 marks

(0.5 mark for each correct stem, with a maximum of 3 marks)

Related to vascular access:

- Infection.
- Haemorrhage.
- Local structural trauma.
- Air embolus.

Reactions to the replacement fluid:

- Transfusion reactions (e.g. febrile reactions, allergic reactions, anaphylaxis, ABO incompatibility).
- Hypothermia (if cold replacement fluid infused at speed).
- Coagulopathy.

- Suxamethonium apnoea (as the plasma cholinesterase has been plasmapheresed off).

References

1.   Yuki N, Hartung HP. Guillain-Barré syndrome. *N Engl J Med* 2012; 366: 2294-304.

Electrocardiography — set 1

1) This is an electrocardiogram (ECG) of a 76-year-old man who has been admitted with abdominal pain for which he is about to undergo an emergency laparotomy (● Figure 1.13). Please describe this ECG.

4 marks
(0.5 mark for each correct stem)

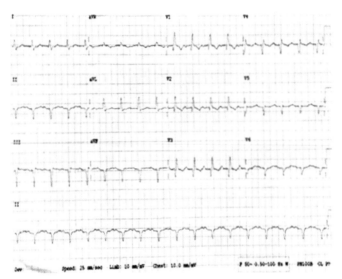

Figure 1.13.

- Rate — 100 beats per minute (bpm) (you need to be within 10 beats per minute of the answer for the mark).
- Rhythm — sinus rhythm (SR).
- Axis — left axis deviation (you may be asked to attempt a rough calculation of the axis, in this case approximately 45°).

- P-wave morphology and P-R interval — normal P-wave, prolonged P-R interval.
- QRS complex — broad complex.
- ST segments — isoelectric.
- T-wave morphology — T-wave inversion V1-V4.
- Other overall comments — right bundle branch block (RBBB).

2) What is the diagnosis?   1 mark

- 1st degree heart block, left axis deviation, RBBB. This is trifascicular block.

3) How would you manage this patient?   1 mark

- Referral for cardiology review as this patient may need a pacing modality instituted prior to surgery.

4) This ECG belongs to an 85-year-male with known ischaemic heart disease, who has

4 marks

(0.5 mark for each correct stem)

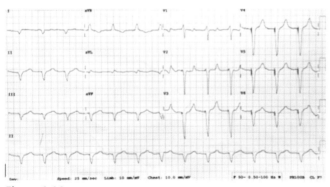

Figure 1.14.

presented with a fractured neck of the femur
(● Figure 1.14). Please describe this ECG.

- Rate — 90 bpm.
- Rhythm — sinus rhythm (SR). Pacing spikes in V2-V6.
- Axis — left axis deviation (approximately -110°).
- P-wave morphology and P-R interval — normal P-wave morphology, prolonged P-R.
- QRS complex — broad complex.
- ST segments — isoelectric.
- T-wave morphology — normal T-waves.
- Bundle branch block — cannot comment as paced.

5) What is the diagnosis?   1 mark

- Paced rhythm.

6) What steps would you take before this man   1 mark
went to the operating theatre?

- Arrange for an electrophysiologist from the cardiology department to carry out a pacemaker check.

7) This ECG belongs to a 74-year-old female with   4 marks
diabetes mellitus, who has presented with   (0.5 mark for
chest pain (● Figure 1.15). Please describe this   each correct
ECG.   stem)

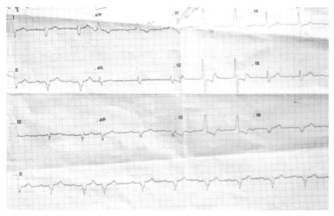

Figure 1.15.

- Rate — 60bpm.
- Rhythm — sinus rhythm (SR).
- Axis — left axis (approximately -110°).
- P-wave morphology and P-R interval — normal morphology, prolonged PR.
- QRS complex — broad.
- ST segments — ST depression seen in V2, V3 (but note cannot comment with bundle branch block).
- T-wave morphology — T-wave inversion V1.
- Bundle branch block? — right bundle branch block (RBBB).
- Note Q-waves in II, III aVF.

8) What is the diagnosis? 2 marks

- RBBB with evidence of an old inferior infarct.

9) How would you manage this patient?   2 marks

- Acute assessment, resuscitation and management should be undertaken to follow an 'airway, breathing, circulation, disability and exposure' approach.
- Cardiology referral with a view to revascularisation.

Radiology — set 1

1) This is a CT scan from a 23-year-old gentleman who was involved in a road traffic accident (Figure 1.16). What does this CT scan show?

3 marks

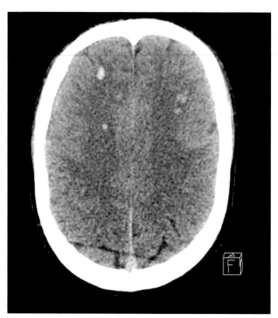

Figure 1.16.

- Loss of grey/white differentiation.
- Small intraparenchymal haemorrhages.
- Loss of sulci.

2) What is the diagnosis?   1 mark

• Diffuse axonal injury.

3) What possible complication of this injury most   2 marks
    concerns you?

• Brain oedema leading to raised intracranial pressure
   (ICP).

4) The following CT is obtained on a 73-year-old   4 marks
    female who was found collapsed at home (●
    Figure 1.17). What does this CT show?

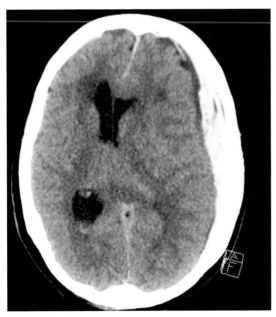

Figure 1.17.

- There is a large left-sided subdural bleed.
- A significant midline shift to the right.
- The left lateral ventricles are effaced.
- Dilatation of the right lateral ventricle.

5) How would you manage this patient?   3 marks

- Acute assessment, resuscitation and management should be undertaken to follow an 'airway, breathing, circulation, disability and exposure' approach.
- Medical management of raised ICP.
- Urgent neurosurgical opinion.

6) The following CT was obtained from an 80-year-old patient who presented with seizures (● Figure 1.18). What does this CT show?   2 marks

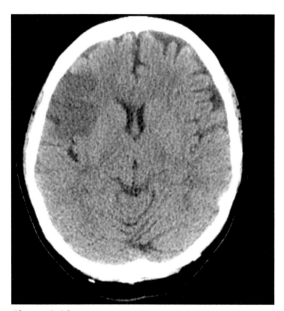

Figure 1.18.

- A right MCA territory infarct.

7) What complication is this patient at risk of?   1 mark

- Malignant middle cerebral artery (MCA) syndrome.

8) What is the pathophysiology of this condition?   2 marks

- Oedema surrounding the original infarct leading to raised intracranial pressure and further compromise to cerebral perfusion.

9) Are you aware of any treatments for this condition and is there any evidence for them?   2 marks

- Decompressive hemicraniectomy.
- Seven randomised controlled trials all show an improvement in mortality; however, many patients are left with significant morbidity.

References

1. Rangel-Castillo L, Gopinath S, Robertson CS. Management of intracranial hypertension. *Neurologic Clinics* 2008; 26(2): 521-41.

2. Dinsmore J. Traumatic brain injury: an evidence-based review of management. *Cont Educ Anaesth Crit Care Pain* 2013; 13(6): 189-95.

Chapter 2

Capnography

You are the doctor on the ICU. A nurse looking after a 32-year-old male who is being mechanically ventilated asks for your advice regarding his ventilator settings.

1) You are presented with the following waveform (● Figure 2.1). What is this waveform?   1 mark

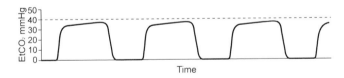

Figure 2.1.

● This is an end-tidal CO_2 trace or capnography trace.

2) Please describe the waveform.   4 marks

(1 mark for each correct stem)

There are different phases to the waveform which are as follows:

- Phase I (inspiratory baseline) reflects inspired gas, which is normally devoid of CO_2.
- Phase II (expiratory upstroke) is the transition between VDana, which does not participate in gas exchange, and alveolar gas from the respiratory bronchioles and alveoli.
- Phase III is the alveolar plateau. Traditionally, PCO_2 of the last alveolar gas sampled at the airway opening is called the $ETCO_2$.
- Phase 0 is the inspiratory downstroke, the beginning of the next inspiration.

3) Which point represents end-tidal CO_2?   0.5 mark

- The highest point of the plateau phase.

4) Which is higher — end-tidal CO_2 or arterial CO_2?   0.5 mark

- Arterial CO_2 is higher than end-tidal CO_2.

5) You are now presented with the following waveform (● Figure 2.2). Please describe the following waveform.   2 marks

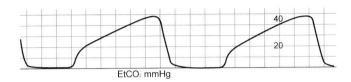

EtCO₂ mmHg

Figure 2.2.

- There is a flattening of the expiratory upstroke and a loss of the plateau phase.

6) What may have caused this?   1 mark

- Asthma or bronchospasm.

7) Despite treatment he continues to deteriorate   1 mark
   and you see the following trace (● Figure 2.3).
   Please describe this trace.

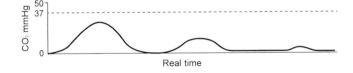

Real time

Figure 2.3.

- There is a decrease in end-tidal CO_2 over a short space of time.

8) What could have caused this?

3 marks

(0.5 mark for each correct stem)

- A decrease in cardiac output, such as cardiac arrest, hypotension, cardiogenic shock.
- A V/Q mismatching, such as in a massive pulmonary embolus.
- An interference with gas exchange, such as pulmonary oedema (though this is unlikely in the above trace).
- A problem with equipment, for example, capnograph failure or a sample line being kinked.
- A blockage of the circuit, anywhere from the endotracheal tube to the ventilator.
- An endotracheal tube cuff leak.

9) How would you manage this situation?

4 marks

(1 mark for each correct stem)

- Acute assessment, resuscitation and management should be undertaken to follow an 'airway, breathing, circulation, disability and exposure' approach.
- 100% oxygen.
- Disconnect from the ventilator and use a Mapleson C circuit. Check you can ventilate and assess lung compliance.
- If there is no pulse start chest compressions.

10) What is this trace (Figure 2.4)?   1 mark

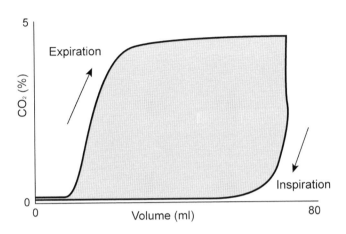

Figure 2.4.

- This is a CO_2 volume trace or volumetric capnography trace.

11) How is it useful?   2 marks

(0.5 mark for each correct stem)

- Gives ventilation/perfusion information.
- Can provide dead space measurement.
- Can provide data on CO_2 elimination.
- Mixed expired CO_2 concentration.

Top Tip

Many of the OSCE stations on equipment or procedures follow topical, current or seminal guidelines. This station was likely to have been triggered due to the importance placed upon the role of end-tidal CO_2 monitoring from the National Audit Project 4 (NAP4) published by The Royal College of Anaesthetists in 2011 [1]. NAP4 highlighted many important aspects of airway management in the critically unwell patient in both the ICU and emergency department setting.

It is important to be familiar with current or seminal guidelines relevant to intensive care, for example, Difficult Airway Society guidelines, Intensive Care Society guidelines and National Institute for Health and Care Excellence (NICE) guidelines.

References

1.   Cook T, Woodall N, Frerk C; The Royal College of Anaesthetists. 4th National Audit Project (NAP 4). The Royal College of Anaesthetists, 2011.

Hepatic failure and ascitic tap

A 57-year-old music journalist is referred to critical care with a low GCS of 4/15. The gentleman is known to the hepatology team and had been admitted under their care for the previous 14 days. He was diagnosed with liver cirrhosis related to excess alcohol 1 year prior to this current admission. On that occasion the patient had decompensated liver failure precipitated by variceal bleeding. He required endoscopic-guided banding and critical care intervention. He survived that episode. He proceeded to abstain from alcohol for 8 months; however, he has recently begun drinking again. This led to this current admission. The patient has gross ascites and has had 1.5L drained during this admission. Despite medical treatment the patient has deteriorated over a 24-hour period with a decreasing conscious level.

1) Please summarise the blood tests below (● Table 2.1).

Table 2.1. Blood test results.	
Hb	89g/L
WCC	19×10^9/L
Platelets	98×10^9/L
Neutrophils	17×10^9/L
INR	3.2
Cl⁻	92mmol/L
HCO₃⁻	19mmol/L
Bilirubin	92µmol/L

Continued overleaf

Table 2.1. Blood test results *continued*.

ALP	125i.u./L
AST	89i.u./L
GGT	320i.u./L
Albumin	22g/L
Amylase	42i.u./L

- Anaemia. — 0.5 mark
- Neutrophilia and raised white cell count. — 0.5 mark
- Evidence of hepatocellular liver damage — liver biochemical derangements, raised bilirubin, raised GGT. — 1 mark
- Synthetic function of liver dysfunctional — characterised by a raised INR and low albumin. — 1 mark

2) His team have performed an arterial blood gas. Please summarise the results below (● Table 2.2). — 1 mark

Table 2.2. Arterial blood gas results.

Face mask FiO$_2$	0.6
pH	6.98
PaO$_2$	8.4kPa
PaCO$_2$	6.0kPa
HCO$_3^-$	16mmol/L
Cl$^-$	92mmol/L
Lactate	3.2mmol/L
BE	-4.2mmol/L

- There is a mixed respiratory and metabolic acidosis.

3) **What immediate management does this patient require?**   3 marks (0.5 mark for each correct stem)

- Acute assessment, resuscitation and management should be undertaken to follow an 'airway, breathing, circulation, disability and exposure' approach.
- Based on his GCS and metabolic state, intubation and ventilation are required.
- Fluid resuscitation.
- Central access and invasive arterial blood pressure monitoring.
- Septic screen.
- This screen should include blood cultures, urine, and an ascitic tap.

4) **The patient is transferred to the ICU. A septic screen to include an ascitic tap is planned. Describe the process of carrying out an ascitic tap.**

- Obtain consent from the patient or their proxy.   0.5 mark
- Examine the patient clinically to ascertain the most favourable position for a tap (classically using percussion of the abdomen to ascertain the fluid level) and/or use ultrasound to identify the safest, most favourable position.   0.5 mark
- Position the patient, either supine or in the lateral decubitus position, favouring the side where you intend to insert the needle.   0.5 mark
- Ensure full asepsis to include sterile gown gloves and a facemask. Clean the skin thoroughly with chlorhexidine solution, drape the area and also the ultrasound (US) probe.   0.5 mark

- Infiltrate the skin with lidocaine. Insert a 20G needle with a 20ml syringe attached at your chosen site perpendicular to the skin or under US guidance. As you advance your needle slowly, aspirate intermittently until you get fluid return.   1 mark

- Once flow is obtained collect 40ml for tests and cultures.   1 mark

5) What tests should the ascitic fluid be sent for?

3 marks
(0.5 mark for each correct stem, with a maximum of 3 marks)

- Cell count and differential.
- Microscopy, culture and sensitivity (MC&S).
- LDH.
- Albumin.
- Amylase.
- Glucose.
- Cytology.

6) How would you diagnose spontaneous bacterial peritonitis on the basis of the test results?

1 mark

- Polymorphonuclear cells (PMN) of >250 PMNs/mm^3.

7) How would this differ in tuberculosis ascites?

1 mark

- There would be a large cell count of mainly lymphocytes instead of PMNs.

8) The patient has an ascitic white cell count (WCC) of 1800 x 10^9/L. A diagnosis of spontaneous bacterial peritonitis (SBP) is made and the patient is commenced on piperacillin-tazobactam. What further investigations would you consider?

1 mark
(0.5 mark for each correct stem)

- Renal biochemistry.
- Abdominal ultrasound.

9) The patient has an abdominal ultrasound. This reveals a liver with severe cirrhosis, and no evidence of hepatocellular carcinoma or portal vein thrombosis. The kidneys appear normal. The patient has a baseline creatinine of 74μmol/L, which is now 220μmol/L, and the patient's vasopressor requirements continue to increase. The acidosis continues to worsen. What are the likely causes of the acute kidney injury?

2 marks
(0.5 mark for each correct stem)

- Pre-renal — hypoperfusion, sepsis, cardiac failure, hepatic failure.
- Intrinsic renal — nephrotoxic drugs.
- Post-renal — renal outflow obstruction.
- Hepatorenal syndrome.

10) A diagnosis of type I hepatorenal syndrome is made. What is the prognosis of this patient?

1 mark

- Very poor — mortality of 90%.

References

1. http://www.bsg.org.uk/clinical-guidelines/liver/guidelines-on-the-management-of-ascites-in-cirrhosis.html.

2. DellaVolpe JD, Garavaglia JM, Huang DT. Management of complications of end-stage liver disease in the intensive care unit. *J Intensive Care Med* 2014; pii: 0885066614551144.

Compartment syndrome

1) You are presented with the following X-ray (● 2 marks Figure 2.5). Please describe what you see on the X-ray.

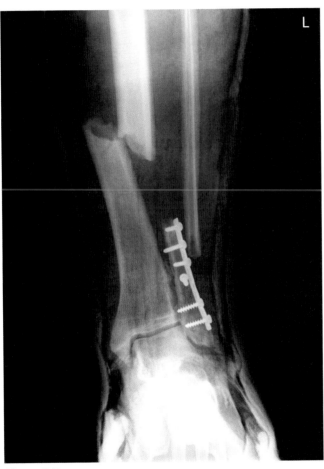

Figure 2.5.

This is a:

- Plain film of the left leg.
- This shows a displaced fracture of both the tibia and fibula.

2) What are the complications of this type of fracture?

3 marks
(1 mark for each correct stem, with a maximum of 3 marks)

- Prolonged healing time.
- Osteomyelitis (especially if it is a compound fracture).
- Nerve injury (peroneal nerve).
- Compartment syndrome.
- Shortened leg length.
- Arthritis.

3) How would you assess the patient for a peroneal nerve injury?

- If the patient is sedated then nerve conduction studies would be required.

1 mark

- If the patient is not sedated and awake then the following clinical features should be looked for:
  - a test of sensation in the dorsum of the foot territory (except between the 1st and 2nd toes);
  - absent ankle jerk;
  - foot drop;
  - muscle strength testing (foot inversion).

2 marks
(0.5 mark for each correct stem, with a maximum of 2 marks)

4) What are the features of compartment syndrome?

3 marks
(0.5 mark for each correct stem)

- Pain which is out of proportion to the injury.
- Paraesthesia.

- Paralysis.
- Pulselessness (late sign).
- Skin changes, tense swollen, shiny skin.
- Venous congestion of the toes with an increased capillary refill time.

5) How would you measure compartment pressures?   2 marks

- A needle attached to a pressure transducer is introduced into the compartment.
- The transducer should be zeroed at the level of the compartment being measured.

6) Label the compartments in the lower limb (●   2 marks
Figure 2.6).   (0.5 mark for each correct stem)

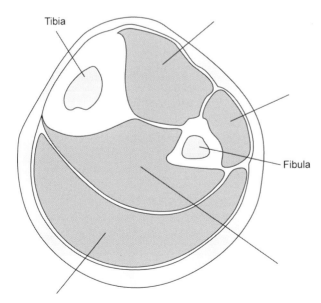

Tibia

Fibula

Figure 2.6.

From the top clockwise the compartments are:

- Anterior.
- Lateral.
- Deep posterior.
- Superficial posterior.

7) What are abnormal compartment pressures?   2 marks

- >30mmHg.
  Or
- >30mmHg difference between the compartment pressure and the diastolic blood pressure.

8) How would you treat this condition and what postoperative complication would you be concerned about?

The patient requires:

- Urgent referral to an orthopaedic surgeon.   0.5 mark
- Fasciotomies.   0.5 mark

The patient is at risk of:

- Rhabdomyolsis.   1 mark
- Acute kidney injury.   1 mark

References

1.   Farrow C, Bodenham A. Acute limb compartment syndromes. *Contin Educ Anaesth Crit Care Pain* 2011; 11(1): 24-8.

Intra-aortic balloon pump

A 64-year-old man presents with crushing chest pain to the emergency department in the hospital.

1) An electrocardiogram is performed (Figure 2.7). Please interpret and summarise the following ECG findings.

2 marks

(all stems must be correctly stated to be awarded the 2 marks)

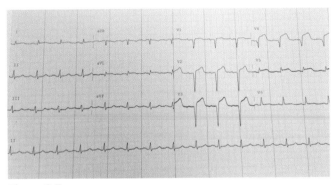

Figure 2.7.

- ST elevation in V2-V4 (anterior leads).
- Some reciprocal changes in the inferior leads II, III and aVF — predominantly in lead III.
- This is an acute ST elevation myocardial infarction in the anterior territory.

2) **What is your immediate management strategy for this patient?**

4 marks (must specify time period for angioplasty and thrombolysis options)

- Acute assessment, resuscitation and management should be undertaken to follow an 'airway, breathing, circulation, disability and exposure' approach.
- Oxygen, aspirin, morphine, nitrates (GTN).
- Revascularisation options:
  - angioplasty for primary percutaneous coronary intervention (PCI) if access is possible within 120 minutes of the time when fibrinolysis could have been given;
  - thrombolysis should be offered if primary PCI is not available within 120 minutes. The pharmacological options include thrombolytic drugs — alteplase, reteplase and streptokinase.

3) The patient is transferred to your hospital, which has a centre for primary percutaneous coronary angiography. Post-procedure he is admitted to the ICU, intubated and ventilated, and becomes hypotensive. What are your management strategies? Please explain your rationale.

- Acute assessment, resuscitation and management should be undertaken to follow an 'airway, breathing, circulation, disability and exposure' approach.

1 mark

- Transthoracic echocardiography (TTE), ideally a transoesophageal echocardiogram (TOE), to assess:

1 mark

- left ventricular function;   0.5 mark
- right ventricular function;   0.5 mark
- post-MI complications — such as left   0.5 mark
  ventricular or interseptal haemorrhage or
  aneurysm.
- Vasopressors, inotropic support.   1 mark
- Intra-aortic balloon pump.   1 mark

4) Please explain the mechanism of action of   4 marks
   the intra-aortic balloon pump.   (2 marks for
                                                 each of the
                                                 key principles)
- A balloon placed under fluoroscopic guidance is
  sited distal to the left subclavian artery.
- The balloon inflates during diastole. This causes an
  increase in coronary and cerebral perfusion, which
  in turn causes an increase in myocardial
  oxygenation.
- The balloon deflates at the end of diastole just
  before systole, in a rapid, sharp manner. This
  reduces the aortic pressure thus decreasing
  'afterload' and, hence, decreasing the work of the
  heart.

5) Please identify labels B, C, D and E on the   2 marks
   following trace (● Figure 2.8).   (0.5 mark for
                                                  each correct
                                                  stem)

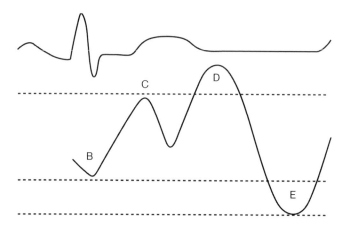

Figure 2.8.

- B — unassisted aortic end-diastolic pressure.
- C — unassisted systolic pressure.
- D — diastolic augmentation.
- E — reduced aortic end-diastolic pressure.

6) Name two complications of an IABP once placed in a patient.

2.5 marks
(0.5 mark for each correct stem, with a maximum of 2.5 marks)

- Ischaemia distally — lower limbs, gut. Hence, there should be vigilance for neurovascular compromise.
- Haemorrhage.
- Haemolysis.
- Thromboembolic phenomenon.

- Balloon rupture.
- Infection.

References

1.   Krishna M, Zacharowski K. Principles of intra-aortic balloon pump counterpulsation. *Contin Educ Anaesth Crit Care Pain* 2009; 9(1): 24-8.

Delirium

You are the doctor on duty for the ICU. Before the ward round the consultant has asked you to assess a gentleman who is on the ICU after a laparotomy for a small bowel perforation. He is currently weaning from the ventilator and has a tracheostomy in place. Last night the nursing staff reported that he was agitated and confused.

In this scenario the patient will be played by an actor with a mock tracheostomy in place.

1) **What scoring systems could you use to assess the patient's confusion?** 1 mark (for either)

- Richmond Agitation Sedation Scale (RASS).
- Ramsey Sedation Scale.

2) **Please assess the patient using the RASS, and explain the process as you assess the patient.** 4 marks

The actor will be asked to simulate a certain RASS score. You will be scored on your assessment as well as a single mark for the correct score.

- Observes the patient.
- Says the patient's name and asks the patient to look at the candidate.
- Correctly scores the patient as -2.

Top Tip

Below is a system for assessing the RASS:

- Observe the patient.
- Assess the patient and classify into one of the following groups:
  - alert and calm (score 0);
  - restless (score +1);
  - agitated (score +2);
  - very agitated (score +3);
  - combative (score +4).

If the patient is NOT alert say the patient's name and ask the patient to open their eyes and look at you. Based on the response, classify into one of the following groups:

- Awakens; sustained eye opening AND eye contact >10 seconds (score -1).
- Awakens; eye opening and eye contact BUT not sustained (score -2).
- Any response to voice but no eye contact (score -3).

If the patient has NO response to verbal stimuli, physically stimulate the patient (e.g. shaking the shoulder or a sternal rub). Based on the response classify into one of the following groups:

- Any movement to stimulation (score -4).
- No response (score -5).

3)   Perform a Confusion Assessment Method for   2 marks
      the Intensive Care Unit (CAM-ICU) score on
      the patient. Candidates will be provided with a
      CAM-ICU checklist (● Figure 2.9) to enable the
      calculation of the score (adapted from Wesley,
      et al. Evaluation of delirium in critically ill
      patients: validation   of   the   Confusion
      Assessment Method for the Intensive Care
      Unit (CAM-ICU). *Crit Care Med* 2001; 29(7):
      1370-9).

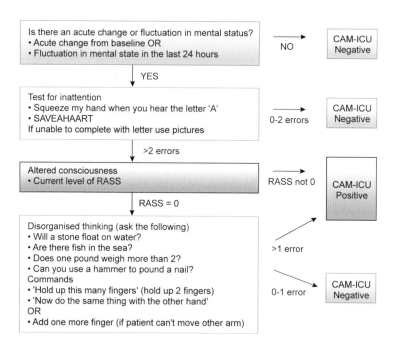

Figure 2.9. CAM-ICU checklist.

The candidate:

- Performs the examination in a systematic manner.
- Correctly scores the patient.

4) What is delirium? 1 mark

- Disturbance of consciousness with a change in cognition that develops over a short time period.

5) How would you classify ICU delirium? 2 marks

(all stems must be correctly stated to be awarded the 2 marks)

- Hyperactive delirium.
- Hypoactive delirium.
- Mixed.

6) What are the risk factors for ICU delirium? 4 marks

(1 mark for each main subgroup with correct example and 1 extra mark for 2 additional examples)

Patient factors:

- Advancing age.
- Depression.
- Alcoholism.
- Hypertension.
- Smoking.
- Visual/hearing impairment.
- Cognitive impairment.

Illness factors:

- Anaemia.
- Acidosis.
- Metabolic disturbances.

- Hypotension.
- Sepsis.

Iatrogenic factors:

- Sleep deprivation.
- Immobilization.
- Medication.

7) How would you manage ICU delirium?

4 marks

(1 mark for each correct stem, with a maximum of 4 marks)

- Address risk factors.
- Sedation holds.
- Attempt to correct sleep-wake cycle.
- Patient orientation.
- Use of visual/hearing aids.
- Medication (as last resort).

8) Why is ICU delirium important?

2 marks

(0.5 mark for each correct stem, with a maximum of 2 marks)

- Increased mortality.
- Increased number of days on a ventilator.
- Increased length of ICU stay.
- Increased incidence of long-term cognitive impairment.
- Increased incidence of adverse events, e.g. self-extubation.

References

1. Brummel NE, Girard TD. Preventing delirium in the intensive care unit. *Crit Care Clin* 2013; 29(1): 51-65.

Infective endocarditis

A 51-year-old woman is admitted to hospital with a 1-day history of sudden-onset bilateral hearing loss and unsteadiness, having been unwell for a few days with general flu-like symptoms. The patient has no relevant past medical or drug history, but is known to have been a previous intravenous drug user. On admission she is found to be pyrexial and tachycardic, with nystagmus and a profound bilateral sensorineural deafness.

1) The following blood test results are obtained (● Table 2.3). Please summarise the blood results.

1 mark
(0.5 mark for each correct stem)

Table 2.3. Blood test results.

Hb	128g/L
WCC	14 x 10^9/L
Platelets	220 x 10^9/L
INR	1.1
Cl$^-$	92mmol/L
HCO$_3^-$	29mmol/L
Bilirubin	14μmol/L
Urea	6.4mmol/L
Creatinine	74μmol/L
CRP	316mg/L
Amylase	14i.u./L
Troponin	>2000ng/L

- Inflammatory markers are raised — WCC and CRP.
- Troponin is significantly raised.

2) An electocardiogram is performed (● Figure 2.10). Please present this ECG.

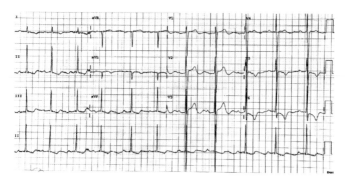

Figure 2.10.

- ST depression in the inferior leads (II, III, aVF).   0.5 mark
- T-wave inversion in the lateral leads (V5, V6, I, aVL).   0.5 mark
- Ischaemic changes.   1 mark

3) The patient suffers a tonic-clonic seizure which is self-limiting after 30 seconds. Based on the history thus far what further investigations would you now request? Please explain your reasoning.

    5 marks
    (1 mark for each correct investigation with correct justification)

- CT head — neurological events including seizure.

- MRI of head and spine — deafness and nystagmus due to a vasculitic process.
- Lumbar puncture — rule out central nervous system infection — meningitis or encephalitis.
- Transthoracic echocardiogram — ECG changes with rise in troponin, to rule out ischaemic causes.
- Further laboratory tests to include ESR, auto-antibody screen — other vasculitic causes.

4) A lumbar puncture is performed. The results are detailed below (● Table 2.4). Summarise the lumbar puncture results and suggest a differential diagnosis.

2 marks
(1 mark for each correct stem)

Table 2.4. Lumbar puncture results.

Protein	0.2g/L
WCC	336/mm^3
Lymphocytes	90%
RCC	2/mm^3
Glucose	2mmol/L
Fluid appears discoloured but not frankly turbid	

- Raised WCC — it is predominantly lymphocytic, therefore, it could be mycobacterial tuberculosis or a fungal infection.
- However, a bacterial cause cannot be ruled out.

5) The patient has been placed on broad- 1 mark
spectrum antibiotic therapy and an infective
cause is sought. A decision is made to further
investigate with echocardiography. What form
of echocardiography is the most sensitive for
detecting endocarditis?

- Transoesophageal echocardiography (TOE).
- TOE has a sensitivity of 90% whereas TTE has a
  sensitivity of 50%.

6) What potential problems are posed by TOE? 1 mark

- This is an invasive test and as such it requires sedation
  or anaesthesia.

Potential complications include: 1 mark

(for any 2

- Oesophageal injury (including perforation). complications)
- Gastric injury.
- Displacement of the endotracheal tube.

Top Tip

Echocardiography images are becoming increasingly common in
ICU exams. It is well worth spending some time familiarising
yourself with the common TTE and TOE views.

7) The TTE and a further transoesophageal echocardiogram confirm that vegetations are seen on the mitral valve causing significant mitral regurgitation. A blood culture from admission has grown *Staphylococcus aureus*. A diagnosis of infective endocarditis (IE) is made. Are you aware of any diagnostic system for infective endocarditis?

1 mark

- Duke criteria or modified Duke criteria.

Should the candidate fail to identify the Duke criteria, please ask them directly.

8) What are the modified Duke criteria?

- There are major and minor criteria. 1 mark
- A diagnosis of IE can be made based on having one of the three following permutations:
  - 2 major criteria;
  - 1 major criteria and 3 minor criteria;
  - 5 minor criteria.

1 mark
(for 2 correct permutations)

The criteria are outlined in ● Table 2.5.

4 marks
(1 mark for each correct major criteria definition, and 0.5 mark for each minor criteria definition)

Table 2.5. Duke major and minor criteria.

Major criteria

- Positive blood culture (BC) for IE:
  - two separate BCs with a typical organism, for example, *Streptococci viridans* or *Staphylococcus aureus*.
- Echocardiogram indicative of IE:
  - oscillating mass on valve or endocardial structures with equivalent regurgitant jets or alterations in anatomy;
  - prosthetic valve disruption;
  - intracardiac abscess.

Minor critieria

- Fever >38°C.
- Intravenous drug use or preexisting cardiac condition which could predispose to IE.
- BC and echocardiographic findings which could be IE but do not meet the precise major criteria definition.
- Peripheral examination for immunological stigmata of IE — Janeway lesions, Osler's nodes, splinter haemorrhages.

Top Tip

See below for lumbar puncture interpretation of results.

- Normal:
  - pressure 5-20cm H_2O;
  - appearance is normal;
  - protein 0.18-0.45g/L;
  - glucose 2.5-3.5mmol/L;
  - Gram stain is normal;
  - glucose — CSF: serum ratio 0.6;
  - WCC <3/mm^3.

- Bacterial:
  - pressure >30cm H_2O;
  - appearance is turbid;
  - protein >1g/L;
  - glucose <2.2mmol/L;
  - Gram stain is 60-90% positive;
  - glucose — CSF: serum ratio <0.4;
  - WCC >500/mm^3;
  - 90% PMN.

- Viral:
  - pressure is normal or mildly increased;
  - appearance is clear;
  - protein <1g/L;

- glucose normal;

- Gram stain is normal;

- glucose — CSF: serum ratio >0.6;

- WCC <1000/mm^3;

- Monocytes 10% have >90% PMN; 30% have >50% PMN.

- Fungal/TB:

  - appearance of fibrin web;

  - protein 0.1-0.5g/L;

  - glucose 1.6-2.5mmol/L;

  - glucose — CSF: serum ratio <0.4;

  - WCC 100-500/mm^3;

  - Monocytes.

References

1.   Eleftherios M, Calderwood SB. Infective endocarditis in adults. *New Engl J Med* 2001; 345(18): 1318-30.

Disseminated malignancy

You are asked to review a 49-year-old homeless man in the emergency department. He was brought in by ambulance having been found unconscious by the police. He has been in the emergency department for the last 30 minutes and the doctor in the department has called you as they are concerned that he appears to be having difficulty breathing.

1) Please outline your initial management.

2 marks

(all stems must be correctly stated to be awarded the 2 marks)

- Acute assessment, resuscitation and management should be undertaken to follow an 'airway, breathing, circulation, disability and exposure' approach.
- Ensure high-flow oxygen via a non-rebreathe bag.
- Check airway patency.

2) He has a Glasgow Coma Scale (GCS) of 15/15 and is talking to you in sentences. What would be your next priority?

1 mark

- Obtain a set of observations.
- Establish IV access and send for blood tests.

3) What blood tests would you send for?

2 marks

(all stems must be stated to be awarded the marks)

- Full blood count.
- Urea and electrolytes.
- Liver biochemistry.
- CRP.
- Coagulation screen.

4)   What other tests would you request?   3 marks

- Urinary antigens for *Pneumococcus* and *Legionella*.
- Sputum sample if possible.
- Chest X-ray.

5)   Here is his chest X-ray (● Figure 2.11). What are your differential diagnoses?

2 marks

(0.5 mark for each correct stem or substem)

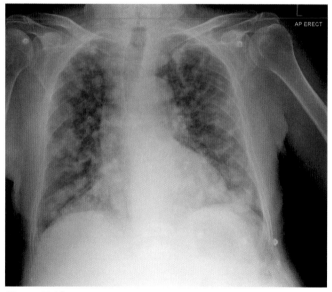

Figure 2.11.

- Malignancy.
- Other infection — viral, bacterial, protozoal or fungal:
  - *Pneumocystis jirovecii;*
  - tuberculosis.
- Interstitial lung disease.

- Inflammatory or autoimmune disease, for example, sarcoidosis.

6) You receive the following blood results (● Table 2.6). Summarise the abnormalities.

3 marks

Table 2.6. Blood test results.	
Hb	135g/L
WCC	11.4 x 10^9/L
Platelets	313 x 10^9/L
Na$^+$	142mmol/L
K$^+$	4.3mmol/L
Total bilirubin	32µmol/L
Urea	8.9mmol/L
Creatinine	110µmol/L
Albumin	28g/L
Total ALP	78i.u./L
ALT	124i.u./L
GGT	203i.u./L

There is:

- A high white cell count.
- A low albumin level.
- An abnormal set of liver biochemistry, characterised by raised gamma-glutamyl transpeptidase (GGT) and alanine aminotransferase (ALT).

7) What further tests would you request?

3 marks
(1 mark for each correct stem)

- CT of the chest.
- Ultrasound or CT of the abdomen.
- Tumour markers (CA19-9, CEA).

8) A CT scan reveals a large intra-abdominal mass associated with the head of the pancreas, as well as multiple lytic lesions in the thoracic vertebrae. What is the pathology exhibited in the chest X-ray?

1 mark

- Lymphangitis carcinomatosis.

9) How would you manage this patient?

3 marks
(1 mark for each correct stem)

- This patient may not be appropriate for admission to critical care.
- In view of disseminated malignancy, the case requires discussion between the relevant teams involved in the patient's care, prior to a decision to admit to critical care.
- Involvement of the patient and next of kin is crucial in discussion regarding ongoing treatment.

Professionalism — failed discharge

You are the on-call doctor for the ICU. The nurse in charge of the unit has asked you to talk to the daughter of a recently admitted patient.

He is a 78-year-old man who was discharged from the unit the previous day after a 10-day admission for a community-acquired pneumonia. He has a past medical history of ischaemic heart disease and chronic obstructive airway disease. Overnight he decompensated on the ward and required readmission to the ICU.

His daughter has asked to speak to the medical staff to explain the events overnight.

This station will have an actress playing the part of the daughter.

1) Please discuss the case with the daughter and outline the first step with regard to this incident.   2 marks

The candidate:

- Provides an appropriate introduction, including their name, grade and role.
- Establishes the nature of the relative's enquiry.

2) The patient's daughter is upset and angry. She asks why her father was discharged only to

need readmitting. She becomes tearful as she explains the stress of the past 2 weeks.

The candidate:

- Allows the relative to talk without interruption, establishing her concerns. 2 marks
- Uses open questions and listens sympathetically. 1 mark

3) The relative explains that she now has no faith in the care on the ward and will not let her father be cared for in any environment other than critical care. 2 marks

The candidate:

- Explains to the relative that this is not feasible, but that they will ensure that the patient is not discharged until he is safe for ward care.

4) At this point the relative becomes angry and agitated, saying "well it didn't work last time did it!" 3 marks

The candidate:

- Reassures the relative that there are systems in place to ensure the safety of recently discharged patients.
- Mentions the critical care outreach service or review by a colleague post-discharge.

5) The relative calms down when these services are outlined. She now asks "how can these events be prevented from happening again?"

The candidate:

- Informs the relative of the critical incident reporting system.   1 mark
- Informs the relative of the following: 5 marks
    - a report of the incident will be created;
    - it will be investigated by the trust;
    - the risk of it occurring again will be graded;
    - the trust will then put in place systems to prevent it occurring again;
    - they will be informed of the progression of the investigation of the incident.

6) The relative tells the candidate the she blames a nurse on the ward, who she feels didn't look after her father correctly.   2 marks

The candidate:

- Offers to allow the relative to meet with the ward nurse to discuss her concerns.
- Suggests that on discharge the patient could be placed on an alternative ward.

7) The relative marks the candidate on the following: 2 marks

- Empathetic.
- Communicated effectively, and without jargon.

Lumbar puncture

You are the doctor on the ICU and have been asked to perform a lumbar puncture on a 63-year-old patient who was recently admitted in septic shock with a low GCS. You may assume valid consent has been obtained.

In this station there will be a manikin and appropriate equipment for the candidate to use.

1) **Please demonstrate on the manikin how you would perform a diagnostic lumbar puncture. You will be asked questions at the end of the procedure.**

7 marks (1 mark for each correct stem, with a maximum of 7 marks)

The candidate should demonstrate and verbally clarify that they are carrying out the following steps:

- Uses aseptic technique.
- Positions the patient appropriately.
- Cleans the skin with chlorhexidine, which is allowed to dry.
- Uses local anaesthesia.
- Demonstrates assessing appropriate level for needle insertion.
- Inserts the needle into the manikin and obtains 'cerebrospinal fluid' (CSF).
- Obtains a manometer reading of the opening pressure.
- Takes four samples (numbered) and a glucose sample.

2) What test would you send the samples for?

4 marks
(1 mark for each correct stem, with a maximum of 4 marks)

- Microscopy, cell count and culture.
- Viral polymerase chain reaction (PCR).
- Protein (oligoclonal bands).
- Glucose.
- Xanthochromia.

3) What are the indications for lumbar puncture?

2 marks
(0.5 mark for each correct stem)

- Diagnosis of subarachnoid haemorrhage.
- Diagnosis of meningitis/encephalitis.
- To aid with the diagnosis of other central nervous system diseases such as Guillain-Barré syndrome.
- Therapeutic relief of benign intracranial hypertension.

4) List the contraindications of lumbar puncture.

2 marks
(0.5 mark for each correct stem)

- Signs of raised intracranial pressure (either clinical or on CT).
- Coagulopathy.
- Localised skin infection.
- Patient refusal.

5) List the complications of lumbar puncture.

3 marks
(0.5 mark for each correct stem)

- Bleeding or haematoma.
- Failure.
- Nerve damage.
- Post-dural puncture headache.
- Infection.
- Dysaesthesia.

6)   You are presented with the following results   2 marks
     (● Table 2.7). What are the abnormalities and
     what is the most likely diagnosis?

Table 2.7. Results of lumbar puncture.

Protein	1.5g/dL
WCC	1200/mm^3
RCC	5/mm^3
Glucose	2mmol/L
Appearance of fluid	Turbid-looking fluid

* There is a raised WCC and high protein levels with a
  low glucose level, along with turbid CSF.
* These are all indicative of bacterial meningitis.

(See the Top Tip on p93 in the 'Infective endocarditis'
OSCE station.)

Local anaesthetic toxicity

An 83-year-old lady has been admitted to hospital having sustained a fall. She has a past medical history of hypertension and has been losing weight over the last 2 years, now weighing 40kg, but is otherwise fit and healthy. The fall is believed to have been mechanical in nature. The patient has the following image at admission (Figure 2.12), and is prescribed 1g of paracetamol and 5mg of morphine. Routine blood tests are carried out.

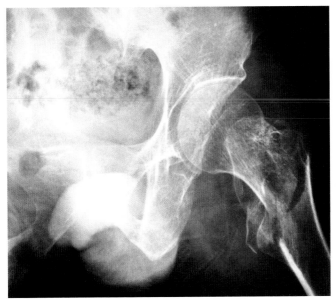

Figure 2.12.

1) Please present the abnormal findings on this X-ray.   1 mark

- Left-sided subcapital impacted fractured neck of the femur.

- Otherwise, the bony structures look intact, with no other pathology to note.

2) You are the intensive care doctor on-call and are called as part of the cardiac arrest team. The patient has had a seizure and developed significant cardiovascular instability. Of note the patient had been in significant pain despite the medicines administered. The only other intervention undertaken since admission was when an emergency medicine doctor had successfully placed a fascia iliaca block (FIB) using a landmark technique for analgesia approximately 5 minutes before.

    1 mark

    The following ECG is obtained (Figure ● 2.13). Please summarise this ECG.

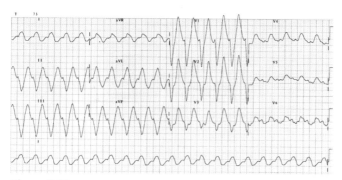

Figure 2.13.

- Broad complex tachycardia — rate of between 120-130 bpm.
- Ventricular tachycardia (VT).

3) What is your plan?

- This is a critical emergency.   0.5 mark
- Acute assessment, resuscitation and management   0.5 mark
  should be undertaken to follow an 'airway, breathing,
  circulation, disability and exposure' approach.
- The neurological sequelae:
  - seizure control;   0.5 mark
  - benzodiazipines   first-line   —   lorazepam   0.5 mark
    0.1mg/kg IV.
- Cardiovascular sequelae:
  - the patient still has a pulse;   0.5 mark
  - measures and preparations for synchronised   0.5 mark
    electrical cardioversion.

4) The patient had a total of 40ml of 0.25%   1 mark
bupivacaine injected as part of the FIB. What is
the likely diagnosis?

- The patient has developed local anaesthetic (LA)
  toxicity.
  Or:
- An overdose of LA or a sodium-channel blocking
  agent.

5) What is the safe amount in millilitres that this   2 marks
patient could have had injected?

- The maximum dose of bupivacaine is 2mg/kg.
  2 times 40kg = 80mg maximum dose.
  80mg
  0.25% = 2.5mg per ml
  80mg divided by 2.5mg = 32ml.

6) You recognise that this is a toxicity related to LA. What are the features of LA toxicity?

Neurological

2 marks

(0.5 mark for each correct stem, with a maximum of 2 marks)

The following is a list of the progression of symptoms:

- Sensorineural — strange tastes, smells, sensations.
- Visual, auditory disturbances.
- Paraesthesia, tingling.
- Agitiation, anxiety, headache.
- Generalised tonic-clonic seizures.
- Loss of consciousness.

Cardiovascular

- The primary cardiac effects of LAs is a decrease in the rate of depolarisation in the fast conducting tissues of the myocardium. This is due to the blockade of Na^+ fast channels.

1 mark

- Prolonged PR.
- QRS widening.
- Prolonged QT.
- Dissemination to ventricular tachyarrhythmias and cardiac arrest.

2 marks

(0.5 mark for each correct stem)

Vascular effects

- LAs may have a biphasic effect. At low concentrations, LAs cause vasoconstriction. At high or toxic concentrations, they cause vasodilation.

1 mark

7) The patient deteriorates further and there are   4 marks
no signs of life. CPR is commenced. What
specific considerations or measures would you
have with regards to the LA toxicity?

- Acute assessment, resuscitation and management
  should be undertaken to follow an 'airway, breathing,
  circulation, disability and exposure' approach.
- CPR may be prolonged — so make the team aware
  of the potential for this.
- Administer Intralipid®.
- Administer sodium bicarbonate.

8) Should CPR be carried out for this patient?   1 mark

- Although this patient is elderly, bearing in mind she is
  otherwise fit and well until this acute iatrogenic insult,
  CPR should be carried out until a formal decision is
  made with the team.

9) What other Na+ channel blocking agents are   1 mark
related with toxicity?

- Tricyclic antidepressants.
- Antiarrhythmic agents, for example, flecainide.

References

1.   http://www.aagbi.org/sites/default/files/la_toxicity_2010_0.pdf.

Electrocardiography — set 2

1) A 52-year-old diabetic man presents to the emergency department. An ECG is recorded (Figure ● 2.14). Please review and then present the findings on this patient's ECG.

3 marks
(0.5 mark for each correct stem, with a maximum of 3 marks)

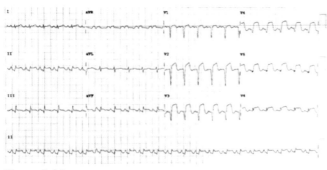

Figure 2.14.

- Rate — 120 bpm (you need to be within 10 beats per minute of the answer for the mark).
- Rhythm — sinus rhythm (SR).
- Axis — normal axis.
- P-wave morphology and P-R interval — normal P-wave, normal P-R interval.
- QRS complex — normal.
- ST segments — ST elevation in V2, V3, V4, V5, V6, II and aVF.
- T-wave morphology — normal.

2) **What is the diagnosis?**   1 mark

- There is a large ST elevation MI in the anterolateral and inferior territories.

3) **How would you manage this patient?**   2 marks

- Acute assessment, resuscitation and management should be undertaken to follow an 'airway, breathing, circulation, disability and exposure' approach.
- Urgent referral for revascularisation.

4) **Please detail the revascularisation options available to you in a small remote hospital.**   2 marks

- If access for percutaneous coronary intervention (PCI) is less than 120 minutes, then this should be undertaken with urgency.
- If access to PCI is greater than 120 minutes, then thrombolysis with recombinant tissue plasminogen activator (r-tPA), for example, alteplase or streptokinase, should be given.

5) **You are asked by a work colleague to comment on the ST elevation seen in V1 and V2 in this ECG (Figure ● 2.15). The patient is stable and well. Please describe the main feature of this ECG and provide a suitable comment for your colleague.**   3 marks
(1 mark for each correct stem, with a maximum of 3 marks)

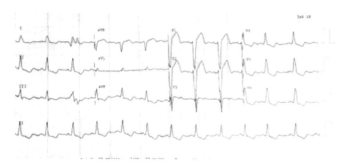

Figure 2.15.

- The patient has left bundle branch block (LBBB).
- Whilst this patient has LBBB the ST segment changes cannot be interpreted.
- The patient may have old ECGs to compare and assess as these changes may be longstanding.
- Concurrently the patient should be assessed for any features of myocardial ischaemia, as new-onset symptomatic LBBB will require referral and review by a cardiologist potentially for revascularisation.

6)   A 69-year old man with end-stage renal failure has this ECG recorded (Figure ● 2.16). Please describe this ECG.

3 marks
(0.5 mark for each correct stem, with a maximum of 3 marks)

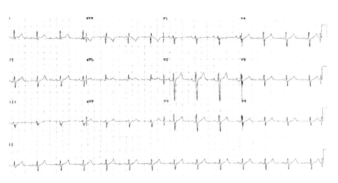

Figure 2.16.

- Rate — 80 bpm (you need to be within 10 beats per minute of the answer for the mark).
- Rhythm — sinus rhythm (SR).
- Axis — left axis deviation.
- P-wave morphology and P-R interval — normal P-wave, slightly prologed P-R interval.
- QRS complex — normal.
- ST segments — ST normal.
- T-wave morphology — peaked T-waves in V2, V3, V4, V5.

7) What is the most likely cause of peaked T-wave morphology in this case?   1 mark

- Hyperkalaemia.

8) How would you manage hyperkalaemia in this patient if the potassium levels read 6.9?   5 marks

(1 mark for each correct stem)

- Acute assessment, resuscitation and management should be undertaken to follow an 'airway, breathing, circulation, disability and exposure' approach.
- Bloods — to include urea and electrolytes, and an arterial blood gas (ABG) to assess potassium and acidosis.
- Electrocardiogram monitoring and non-invasive blood pressure.
- Emergency medical management of hyperkalaemia:
  - management strategies to drive the potassium intracellularly:
    - insulin (rapid-acting insulin, for example, Actrapid) 10-20 units mixed in 50ml of 50% dextrose;
    - salbutamol nebulisers;

- management to stabilise vulnerable membrane surfaces:
  - calcium chloride — 10ml of 10% given intravenously.
- Haemofiltration or haemodialysis.

Radiology — set 2

1) The following CT scan was obtained from a 76-year-old patient who is currently intubated on the ICU (Figure ● 2.17). What does this CT scan show?

3 marks

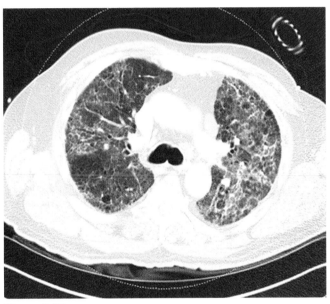

Figure 2.17.

- Bilateral interstitial changes.
- Small bullae.
- Traction bronchiectasis.

2) What is the diagnosis?

1 mark

- Chronic obstructive pulmonary disease (COPD).

3)   What ventilatory strategies would you employ   5 marks
     for this patient?

- Tidal volumes of 6-8ml/kg.
- Allow sufficient expiratory time (e.g. increase I:E ratio).
- Appropriate use of positive end-expiratory pressure (PEEP).
- Avoidance of dynamic hyperinflation and 'gas trapping' (e.g. lowering minute ventilation).
- Use of medication to improve airway obstruction (such as bronchodilators).

4)   What type of image is captured on this scan   1 mark
     (Figure ● 2.18)?

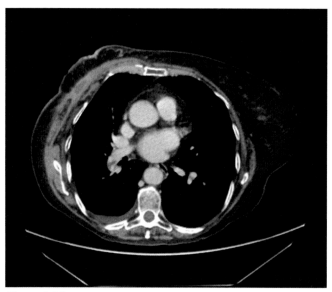

Figure 2.18.

- CT pulmonary angiography.

5) What abnormalities does it show?   1 mark

- A filling defect in the right pulmonary artery, consistent with a pulmonary embolus (PE).

6) Do you know of a classification system for pulmonary embolus?

3 marks
(1 mark for stating and defining sub-massive PE, and 2 marks for stating and defining massive PE)

Sub-massive PE:

- Signs of right ventricular strain but no cardiovascular compromise.

Massive PE:

- Signs of right ventricular dysfunction.
- Systolic blood pressure <90mmHg.
- Needing inotropic support.

7) A 64-year-old woman presents with haemoptysis. What abnormality does this CT scan show (Figure ● 2.19)?

1 mark

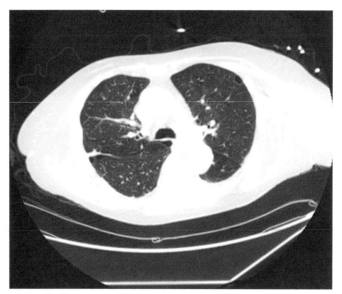

Figure 2.19.

- Cavitating lesions.

8)   **What diagnosis would you consider?**   1 mark

- Tuberculosis.

9)   **What diagnostic tests would you order?**   3 marks

(for any 3
- Sputum for acid-fast bacillus (AFB).   tests)
- Mantoux test.
- Serum tests such as T-Spot or quantiFERON-TB.
- Early morning urine for AFB.

10) How would you treat this patient?

1 mark
(all four stems
must be stated
to be awarded
the mark)

Anti-TB therapy:

- Rifampicin.
- Isoniazid.
- Pyrazinamide.
- Ethambutol.

Chapter 3

Burns

You are the ICU doctor on-call and are called to the emergency department to see a 42-year-old man who was rescued from a house fire. On arrival the patient is self-ventilating on high-flow oxygen through a non-rebreathe mask, he has a **GCS of 14/15** and the emergency department team is gaining intravenous (IV) access.

1) What features specific to this presentation would you need to elicit in your history?

   3 marks
   (0.5 mark for each correct stem)

   - How long ago did the incident occur?
   - What treatment has already been provided?
   - Type of fire — enclosed or open area?
   - Time exposed to heat or fire?
   - Was there significant smoke exposure?
   - Were there any explosions/blast injuries?

2) During your initial assessment, it is apparent that the patient has a mix of erythematous and blistering burn lesions across his face,

   2 marks

with singed eyebrows and eyelashes. The eyes are almost fully closed from the surrounding swelling. What would your first priority be and why?

- The airway requires securing with intubation urgently.
- The airway is likely to swell and if not already compromised is at high risk of compromise.

3) How will you intubate this patient?

3 marks

(0.5 mark for each correct stem)

- Rapid sequence induction.
- Pre-oxygenate.
- Sedative — ketamine, propofol or thiopentone.
- Muscle relaxant — rocuronium or suxamethonium, if less than 12 hours from the burn.
- Cricoid pressure.
- Possible use of opiates.

4) How would you assess the extent of the burns?

2 marks

(0.5 mark for each correct stem)

- Expressed as a percentage of total body surface area (TBSA).
- Use of the Wallace 'rule of 9s' for adults.
- Use of the Lund-Browder charts for both adults and paediatrics.
- The palmar surface of the patient's hand is approximately 1% TBSA.

5) Explain the 'rule of 9s'.

3 marks
(0.5 mark for each correct stem)

- Head is 9%.
- Arms are 9%.
- Legs are 9% anterior and 9% posterior.
- Torso 18%.
- Back 18%.
- Perineum 1%.

6) How would you prescribe fluid in this patient?

3 marks

- Using the Parkland formula which is:

  4ml x percentage total body surface area (TBSA) x the weight in kilograms (kg).

- The first half of this total is given over the first 8 hours, the rest over the next 16 hours.
- Compound sodium lactate is used commonly.

7) What are the risk factors for developing major complications in a burns patient?

2 marks
(1 mark for each correct stem, with a maximum of 2 marks)

- A burn TBSA >40%.
- Age <2 years old or >60 years old.
- Other traumatic injuries.

8) What are some of the complications associated with severe burns?

2 marks
(0.5 mark for each correct stem, with a maximum of 2 marks)

- Hypovolaemia.
- Hypothermia.

- Infection.
- Metabolic abnormalities, e.g. rhabdomyolysis.
- Development of eschars.

References

1. Bishop S, Maguire S. Anaesthesia and intensive care for major burns. *Cont Educ Anaesth Crit Care Pain* 2012; 12(3): 118-22.

Myasthenic crisis

A 71-year-old man requires critical care review in the emergency department having developed progressively worsening dyspnoea, and pooling of secretions at the back of his mouth with visible respiratory distress. Additionally, he reports weakness in his limbs. The patient had a normal CT scan of his head. It transpires that over the last few weeks he had been investigated by his GP for features of diplopia and jaw claudication.

The patient had recently had surgery for prostatic cancer 10 days ago, with a history of ischaemic heart disease.

1) You are presented with the following blood gas results (● Table 3.1). Please summarise the key findings.

1 mark

Table 3.1. Arterial blood gas results.	
Face mask 6L/min approximately an FiO$_2$ 0.4	
pH	7.32
PaO$_2$	12.4kPA
PaCO$_2$	5.9kPA
HCO$_3^-$	28mmol/L
Lactate	1.2mmol/L
BE	+4.9mmol/L
K$^+$	4.6mmol/L

- There is a partially compensated respiratory acidosis.

2) What are the clinical features of concern and what may they indicate in this case?

1 mark
(0.5 mark for each correct stem)

- The respiratory features including dyspnoea and pooling of secretions.
- Indicative of bulbar weakness or palsy.

3) Please list some potential differential diagnoses for this case.

3 marks
(1 mark for each correct stem, with a maximum of 3 marks)

- Cerebrovascular events — ischaemic, haemorrhagic stroke, brainstem (medullary) infarct.
- Neurological condition causing bulbar weakness:
  - inflammatory — Guillain-Barré syndrome;
  - autoimmune — myasthenia gravis;
  - degenerative — motor neurone disease.
- Malignancy — brainstem territory.

4) A neurologist clinically suspects this to be a myasthenic crisis. What is myasthenia gravis and what is the pathophysiology?

3 marks

- An autoimmune disease.
- Antibodies against the post-synaptic nicotinic acetylcholine (Ach) receptors of the neuromuscular junction.
- The low levels of functional Ach receptors cause decreased muscle contraction and, hence, weakness in sustained or repeated activity.

5) List some of the precipitant causes of a myasthenic crisis.

2 marks
(0.5 mark for each correct stem)

- Intercurrent illness.
- Stress.
- Recent surgical intervention/stress.
- Drugs — antibiotics, anticoagulants, anaesthetic agents, cardiac drugs such as beta-blockers.

6) How would you manage this patient's acute state?

- Acute assessment, resuscitation and management should be undertaken to follow an 'airway, breathing, circulation, disability and exposure' approach.   0.5 mark
- Vital capacity (VC) breath assessment.   0.5 mark
- If VC is <20ml/kg, then elective intubation and ventilation are required.   1 mark

7) In a stable patient what specific investigations would you do and what would you be looking for?

- Bedside tests: 0.5 mark
  - VC breath;
  - edrophonium test also known as the Tensilon test.
- Laboratory tests: 0.5 mark
  - autoantibodies against the acetylcholine receptor.
- Radiological: 2 marks
  - CT and/or MRI of the head and chest:
    - rule out intracerebral cause;

- ■ investigate for thymic hyperplasia or thymoma.
- ● Special tests: 1 mark
  - nerve conduction studies;
  - electromyelography.

8) The patient is diagnosed with a myasthenic crisis. What therapeutic measures would you consider, in addition to intubation, ventilation and admission to an ICU?

4 marks
(1 mark for each correct stem, with a maximum of 4 marks)

- ● Anticholinesterases — pyridostigmine.
- ● Immunosuppression — corticosteroids.
- ● Intravenous immunoglobulins (IVIg).
- ● Plasma exchange.
- ● Thymectomy.

References

1.   Spillane J, Higham E, Kullmann D. Myaesthenia gravis. *BMJ* 2012; 345: e8497.

Equipment

1) What is this piece of equipment (● Figure 3.1)?   1 mark

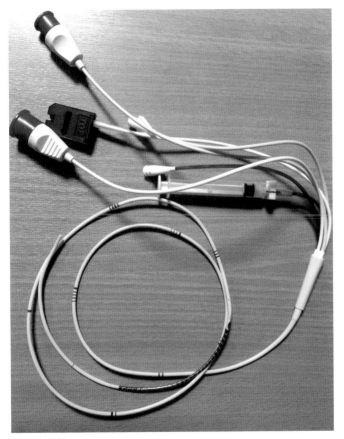

Figure 3.1.

●   This is a pulmonary artery catheter (Swan-Ganz).

2) Please describe the components.　　9 marks

The following parts are identified:

- Two lumens for injecting fluids or drugs — one proximal to the balloon and one distal.
- One lumen with a syringe attached for inflating the balloon. This has an integrated valve.
- Heating coil.
- Balloon just distal to tip.
- Centimetre markings.
- The blue connector is for the optical module allowing mixed venous saturation monitoring.
- Thermal filament.
- Thermistor at 4cm from the tip.
- The red and white connectors — one is for the thermistor and one is for the thermal filament.

3) What measures does this equipment provide?　　4 marks

- Right heart pressures, e.g. right atrial pressure (RAP), pulmonary artery pressures.
- Pulmonary artery occlusion pressure (or 'wedge pressure') which is thought to be equivalent to the left ventricular end-diastolic pressure.
- Cardiac output. The model above allows continuous cardiac output monitoring.
- Mixed venous saturations (SvO_2).

4) How is the cardiac output obtained?　　2 marks

(1 mark for each correct stem, with a maximum of 2 marks)

- Thermodilution.
- Stewart-Hamilton equation.

- Cardiac output is equal to 1/area under curve.

5) **What are the specific complications with pulmonary artery catheters?**

2 marks
(0.5 mark for each correct stem, with a maximum of 2 marks)

- Arrhythmias.
- Valve damage.
- Pulmonary artery (PA) rupture.
- Atrial or ventricular damage, possibly leading to tamponade.
- Knotting of the catheter.
- Thrombus.

6) **Why is SvO_2 greater than $ScvO_2$?**

1 mark

- In health the $ScvO_2$ (central venous saturations) is mainly blood from the superior vena cava (SVC) which consists of blood returning from the brain. This has a higher oxygen extraction ratio, hence the SvO_2 is greater than the $ScvO_2$. However, note in illness, particularly the critically unwell patient, this relationship is not kept as the body in proportion to the disease process extracts more oxygen.

7) **When could pulmonary diastolic pressure be higher than pulmonary wedge pressure?**

1 mark

- In a mechanically ventilated patient if the reading is taken during inspiration the pulmonary diastolic pressure could be higher than the pulmonary wedge pressure.

References

1.   Kelly CR, Rabbani LE. Pulmonary-artery catheterization. *New Engl J Med* 2013; 369(25): e35.

Necrotising fasciitis

A 54-year-old gentleman has a history of diabetes and hypertension, and underwent a recent cholecystectomy for gallstone disease. Subsequent to this, 3 days later, he is admitted to the ICU with features of severe sepsis.

1) The candidate is shown an image (● Figure 3.2). Please describe this image.

2 marks
(0.5 mark for each correct stem, with a maximum of 2 marks)

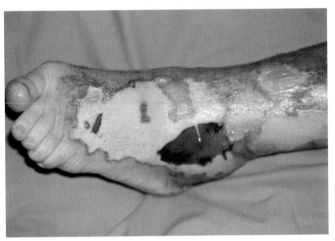

Figure 3.2.

- Anterolateral aspects of the lower leg and foot.
- Widespread rash.
- Areas of erythematous, inflamed regions.
- Areas of black discoloured territory.

- Areas with pealed skin.
- Well-defined borders with some areas of normal tissue.

2) Please list your differential diagnoses.

2 marks
(0.5 mark for each correct stem)

- Trauma — burn injury.
- Reaction — Stevens-Johnson syndrome through to toxic epidermal necrolysis.
- Infection — cellulitis
- Necrotising fasciitis.

3) What is the most likely diagnosis?

0.5 mark

- Necrotising fasciitis.

4) What is necrotising fasciitis and how is this different to cellulitis?

0.5 mark

- It is an infection of the deep fascia and subcutaneous fat unlike cellulitis, which affects the superficial fascia and dermis.

5) Necrotising fasciitis is diagnosed. What are the distinguishing signs and symptoms?

2 marks
(0.5 mark for each correct stem, with a maximum of 2 marks)

- Features of inflammation — erythema, swelling.
- Disproportionate, severe pain.
- Unable to touch the areas due to severity of pain — can appear tense and swollen, with areas of blisters and bullae.

- Features of gangrene — dark discolouration, crepitus can be present in gas-gangrene.
- Systemic features of severe sepsis or septic shock — raised temperature, tachycardia, hypotension.
- The area of involvement can extend and spread rapidly.

6) How would you classify necrotising fasciitis?

Type I:

- Polymicrobial, anaerobic, facultative microorganisms. 0.5 mark
- Affects immunocompromised patients. It can affect the perineum causing Fournier's gangrene. 0.5 mark

Type II:

- Group A beta-haemolytic *Streptococcus*. This can cause the *Streptococcus* toxic shock syndrome. 0.5 mark
- Exotoxin and/or endotoxin release. 0.5 mark

7) How would you manage this patient?

3 marks
(0.5 mark for each correct stem)

- The candidate must state or recognise that this is a critical emergency.
- Acute assessment, resuscitation and management should be undertaken to follow an 'airway, breathing, circulation, disability and exposure' approach.
- Analgesia should be administered as the pain will be severe.
- Septic screen — to include:
  - blood cultures;
  - wound swabs.
- Antibiotics — given early.
- Urgent surgical review — plastic surgical emergency.

8) What specific antibiotics would you consider and why?

2 marks
(0.5 mark for each correct stem)

- High-dose clindamycin which has a potent activity against protein synthesis and, hence, is believed to inhibit toxin production.
- High-dose beta-lactams such as a carbapenem (e.g. meropenem).
- Anaerobic cover with metronidazole.
- If there is septic shock give aminoglycosides.

9) What other useful investigations can be done?

3 marks
(1 mark for each correct stem and an explanation, with a maximum of 3 marks)

- CT.
- MRI.

These imaging modalities help to identify the extent of the condition, evidence of gas gangrene, and may help to guide the level of surgical debridement required.

- Tissue biopsy — distinguishing the tissue diagnosis, for example, between cellulitis and necrotising fasciitis.
- Surgery — during which time surgeons can visually diagnose the extent of the condition and spread.

10) What other management options are available?

3 marks
(1 mark for each correct stem, with a maximum of 3 marks)

- Urgent surgical debridement — may require repeated surgical interventions.
- ICU care organ support as toxic shock could rapidly progress.

- Intravenous immunoglobulins (IVIg).
- Hyperbaric oxygen therapy — particularly for the anaerobic form of necrotising fasciitis.

References

1. Roje Z, Roje Z, Matic D, *et al*. Necrotizing fasciitis: literature review of contemporary strategies for diagnosing and management with three case reports: torso, abdominal wall, upper and lower limbs. *World J Emerg Surg* 2011; 6: 46.

Paracetamol overdose

A 24-year-old female is brought into the emergency department by ambulance after being found collapsed by her boyfriend. She is now registering as 13/15 on the Glasgow Coma Scale (GCS) and is being stabilised prior to being taken for a CT scan of her head.

1) An arterial blood gas (ABG) has been performed and you have been asked to review both the patient and the result, which is included below (● Table 3.2). Please summarise the results.

2 marks

Table 3.2. Arterial blood gas results.

pH	7.15
PaO₂	23.4kPa
PaCO₂	2.3kPa
HCO₃⁻	18.6mmol/L
Lactate	8.6mmol/L
BE	-12mmol/L

- There is a metabolic acidosis and lactataemia.
- Attempted respiratory compensation.

2) What are the differential diagnoses for the acidaemia?

3 marks

(0.5 mark for each correct stem)

- Metabolic disorders.
- Poisoning.

- Ischaemia (characterised by the increasing lactate).
- Acute or chronic renal failure.
- Diabetic emergencies, e.g. diabetic ketoacidosis.
- Diarrhoea.

3) Her blood results are as follows (Table ● 3.3).   2 marks
Please summarise the results.

Table 3.3. Blood test results.	
Hb	113g/L
WCC	5.4×10^9/L
INR	3.4
Na$^+$	135mmol/L
K$^+$	4mmol/L
HCO$_3^-$	18mmol/L
Urea	5.0mmol/L
Creatinine	153μmol/L
ALP	101i.u./L
ALT	900i.u./L
GGT	80i.u./L
Paracetamol	200mg

- Deranged liver biochemistry tests with liver function compromised, as well as characterised by a high INR.
- High paracetamol levels.

4) Please suggest a management plan.

3 marks
(1 mark for each correct stem, with a maximum of 3 marks)

This patient should be managed for acute paracetamol overdose with the following measures and thoughts actively implemented:

- Acute assessment, resuscitation and management should be undertaken to follow an 'airway, breathing, circulation, disability and exposure' approach.
- Supportive treatment.
- No role for activated charcoal in this scenario.
- Intravenous N-acetylcysteine.
- This patient should be managed in a critical care environment.

5) The patient is moved to the ICU and later that evening her GCS drops to 7/15. What are you concerned about and how would you manage the patient?

6 marks
(1 mark for each correct stem, with a maximum of 6 marks)

- This is concerning as it could be a feature of life-critical cerebral oedema.

The management would include:

- Intubation and mechanical ventilation.
- CT scan of the head.
- Measures to lower intracranial pressure (ICP), e.g. conservative — head up 45°, management of PaO_2 and $PaCO_2$.
- Consider ICP monitoring.
- If there are signs of raised ICP, consider osmotic therapy (e.g. mannitol).
- Referral to a tertiary centre.

6) What criteria are you aware of to guide 1 mark
referral for a liver transplant?

- King's criteria.

7) What are the King's criteria for paracetamol- 3 marks
induced liver failure?

- Arterial pH <7.3.

OR all three of the following:

- INR of greater than 6.5.
- Creatinine >300µmol/L.
- Grade III or IV encephalopathy.

Top Tip

For completeness, the King's criteria for non-paracetamol-induced liver failure are:

- INR >6.5 (PT >100 seconds).

OR any three of the following:

- Age <10 or >40 years.
- Aetiology non-A, non-B hepatitis, or idiosyncratic drug reaction.

- Duration of jaundice before hepatic encephalopathy >7 days.
- INR >3.5 (PT >50 seconds).
- Serum bilirubin >300µmol/L (>17.6mg/dL).

It is important to be familiar with the grades of encephalopathy with the West Haven Criteria being the most commonly used system.

- Grade I — Trivial lack of awareness, shortened attention span.
- Grade II — Lethargy or apathy, disorientation.
- Grade III — Somnolence to semistupor, responsive to stimuli.
- Grade IV — Coma.

References

1.   Ferner RE, Dear JW, Bateman DN. Management of paracetamol poisoning. *BMJ* 2011; 342: d2218.

Professionalism — refusal of treatment

You are the doctor on-call for the ICU. You are called upon to speak to a gentleman who has been reviewed by the outreach nurse. The patient has been referred for critical care review for consideration for renal replacement therapy (RRT). The patient was admitted with severe sepsis and managed on the ward with fluid therapy, antibiotics and drainage of an intra-abdominal abscess which was secondary to acute diverticular disease. Although he has made a recovery from the sepsis, particularly following surgical intervention and drainage of the abscess, the patient has suffered an acute kidney injury. The renal function and biochemistry has worsened with creatinine levels at 124μmol/L on admission and now on day 6 of the admission rising without recovery to 524μmol/L. It was agreed that the patient required admission to critical care for renal replacement therapy. The patient has refused renal replacement therapy and has actually wanted to self-discharge himself from the hospital.

In this scenario the patient will be played by an actor.

1) Please discuss the case with the patient and   3 marks
   outline the next steps.

The candidate:

- Provides an appropriate introduction, including their name, grade and role.
- Establishes the identity of the patient, ensuring he is comfortable and offers to have anyone else in the room, for example, a family member or nursing staff.

- Establishes what the patient already knows and understands.

2) The patient is aware he was unwell from a bad infection in his bowel, which has recovered after the surgery and antibiotics. He believes that he can be on oral antibiotics now and that he is much better. He feels a lot better now.

The candidate:

1 mark
(0.5 mark for each correct stem)

- Outlines the clinical events thus far, culminating in the acute kidney injury (AKI) and answers any questions appropriately.
- Informs the patient of the necessity for RRT and describes what RRT is in simple terms.

A schema is detailed below:

- Transfer to a critical care environment (HDU).
- Placing a plastic tube under local anaesthetic into a blood vessel under ultrasound guidance.
- Attaching the tubing to a machine which removes his blood, 'filters' the blood of excess toxins or impurities, before adding in a replacement fluid and infusing back.
- It can be thought of as temporary dialysis.

2 marks
(0.5 mark for each correct stem)

3) The patient is surprised to hear about the problems with his kidneys, but reiterates that he is feeling much better and he understands what has been explained to him and is adamant he does not want any other

2 marks

treatment and wants to be discharged from hospital.

The candidate:

- Appropriately explores the reasons for why the patient wants to be discharged.

4) The patient will eventually reveal that he runs a self-employed family business with many other personal strains and circumstances. **2 marks**

The candidate:

- Is sympathetic to this and takes the time to explore these concerns.
- Explains that without RRT the patient is likely to have worsening medical problems with potentially life-threatening kidney failure.

5) The patient will become impatient and agitated and wants to end the conversation. **3 marks**

The candidate:

- Explains that he or she is duty bound to provide all of the information so that the patient can make an informed decision.
- Explains the severity of the problem in a truthful, concise, yet sympathetic manner.
- Avoids/explains 'jargon'.

6) The patient states that he understands all of this and wants to be discharged.   3 marks

The candidate:

- Explains that you are unable to discharge the patient.
- Offers discussion with seniors (parent team consultant and ICU consultant).
- Explains that if the patient wants to be discharged this will have to be a self-discharge and will be against medical advice.

7) The patient wants to leave immediately and wants the necessary arrangements made.   2 marks

The candidate:

- Explains that he will inform the parent team, the nursing staff and will need to provide paperwork which the patient will need to sign as he is discharging from hospital against medical advice.
- Explains that senior doctors would want to speak with him to ensure that he fully understands the repercussions of not receiving this treatment.

8) The patient accepts all of this and is quite blunt and tells the candidate to make the arrangements quickly or else he will leave without signing anything.   2 marks

- The candidate closes the discussion appropriately.

- On overall review marks are awarded if the candidate communicated in a professional, polite and effective manner.

Top Tip

In these scenarios there are always a number of generic marks for things such as introductions. Don't miss these out!

Pleural effusion

1) Please present the following X-ray (● Figure 3.3).

4 marks
(0.5 mark for each correct stem, with a maximum of 4 marks)

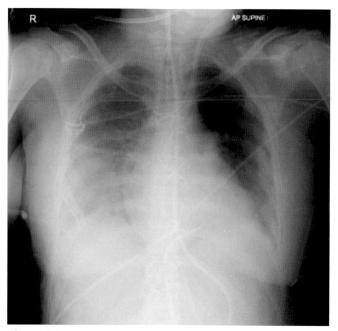

Figure 3.3.

This is an AP chest film. The following features are present:

- Right-sided pleural effusion and/or collapse.
- Nasogastric tube — correctly sited.
- Endotracheal tube — correctly sited.
- Left internal jugular central line and pulmonary artery (PA) catheter sheath.

- Two mediastinal drains.
- Sternal wires.
- Right intercostal drain.
- Pacing wires.
- Electrocardiogram (ECG) electrodes.

2) How would you confirm that this was a pleural effusion?   1 mark

- Ultrasound or CT of the chest.

3) How would you decide whether or not to drain this effusion?   2 marks

- Assess if it is compromising respiratory function; if it is, then an intercostal drain should be inserted.

4) What other reasons might you want to insert an intercostal drain?   1 mark

- If there is suspicion of an underlying pathological process, e.g. malignancy, and if a diagnostic tap is required.

5) How would you determine if the fluid is a transudate or an exudate?   1 mark

- Light's criteria.

6) Can you define Light's criteria?

3 marks

(1 mark for each correct stem)

According to Light's criteria, pleural fluid is an exudate if one of the following is identified from the pleural fluid analysis:

- Ratio of pleural fluid protein to serum protein is >0.5.
- Ratio of pleural fluid lactate dehydrogenase (LDH) to serum LDH is >0.6.
- Pleural fluid LDH is >2/3 times the laboratory's upper limit of a normal range for LDH.

7) List the tests you would request when sending the pleural fluid to the lab.

5 marks

(1 mark for each correct stem, with a maximum of 5 marks)

- Protein.
- LDH.
- Cell count.
- Cytology.
- pH.
- Glucose.
- Cholesterol.
- Amylase.

8) What is the normal pH of pleural fluid?

1 mark

- Pleural fluid has a pH of 7.62.

9) In what pathological conditions will the pleural fluid have a high amylase concentration?

2 marks
(1 mark for each correct stem, with a maximum of 2 marks)

Two out of the following:

- Malignancy.
- Pancreatitis.
- Oesophageal rupture.

Top Tip

The British Thoracic Society (BTS) has quick reference guidelines on many important diseases including asthma, tuberculosis, oxygen therapy and pleural disease. The algorithm overleaf is from the BTS guidelines on pleural disease (● Figure 3.4) [1]. Please refer to the following web site for the full guideline: https://www.brit-thoracic.org.uk/document-library/clinical-information/pleural-disease/pleural-disease-guidelines-2010/pleural-disease-guideline-quick-reference-guide/.

References

1.   British Thoracic Society Pleural Disease Guideline. British Thoracic Society Reports 2010; Vol 2: No 3 (ISSN 2040-2023).

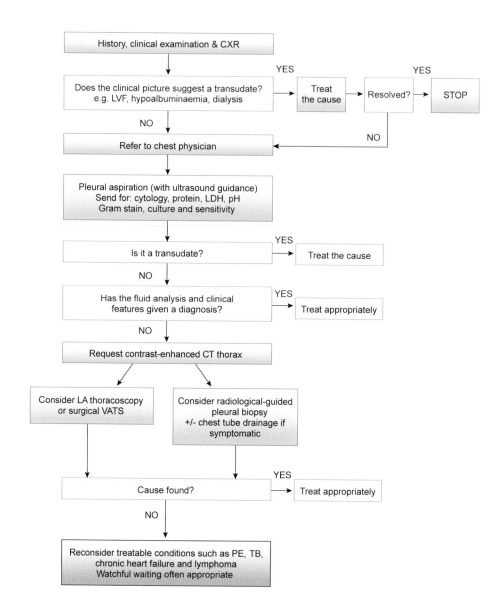

Figure 3.4. British Thoracic Society Pleural Disease Guideline.

Acute respiratory distress syndrome (ARDS)

A 62-year-old man with a body mass index (BMI) of 37 was admitted to hospital with worsening breathlessness. He has a history of being unwell for a few days with non-specific 'flu-like' symptoms.

1) His arterial blood gas (ABG) results are outlined in ● Table 3.4. Please summarise this ABG.

2 marks

Table 3.4. Arterial blood gas results.	
FiO_2	0.8
Hb	113g/L
pH	7.02
PaO_2	8.9kPa
$PaCO_2$	8.7kPa
HCO_3^-	19mmol/L
BE	-5.4mmol/L

- The patient has a severe type II respiratory failure with a PaO_2 of 8.9kPa and a $PaCO_2$ of 8.7kPa.
- There is a mixed respiratory and metabolic acidosis.

2) His conscious level deteriorates rapidly due to fatigue with an acute decline in respiratory effort. Present the key features of this CXR (● Figure 3.5).

2 marks
(0.5 mark for each correct stem, with a maximum of 2 marks)

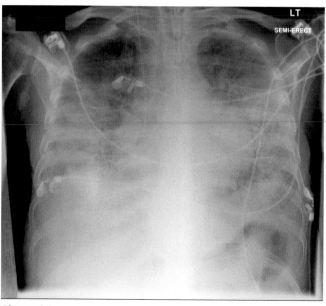

Figure 3.5.

- Right lower lobe consolidation/collapse.
- Bilateral alveolar shadowing.
- This is in keeping with ARDS.
- Central venous line appropriately placed in the right internal jugular vein.
- Endotracheal tube appropriately placed.

3) There is clinical and radiological evidence of acute respiratory distress syndrome (ARDS) and a decision is made to transfer the patient

to the ICU with a view to intubate and ventilate him. Based on the clinical history and rapid deterioration, an empirical diagnosis of community-acquired pneumonia (CAP) complicated by ARDS is made and antibiotics are instituted in accordance with local guidelines for CAP.

What is the Berlin Definition of ARDS?

The Berlin Definition has the following components:

- An acute onset within 1 week or less.   0.25 mark
- Bilateral opacities consistent with pulmonary oedema   0.25 mark must be present and detected on a radiological modality such as CT or a chest radiograph.
- The cause of the alveolar oedema cannot be due to   0.5 mark fluid overload or cardiac failure determined by the clinician's assessment and objective assessment through modalities such as transthoracic echocardiography (TTE) which should be performed if the ARDS does not have a clear-cut cause such as acute pancreatitis, sepsis, burns or trauma.
- ARDS is categorized as being mild, moderate, or   3 marks severe (● Table 3.5).   (1 mark for each correct stem of mild/moderate/ severe categories)

Table 3.5. Categories of ARDS.

ARDS severity	PaO_2/FiO_2	Mortality
Mild	200-300	27%
Moderate	100-200	32%
Severe	<100	45%

- Each category has either a continuous positive airway pressure (CPAP) of 5cmH$_2$O or a positive end-expiratory pressure (PEEP) of 5cmH$_2$O.

4) The patient is intubated and ventilatory support is commenced. Despite a high FiO$_2$ and high inflation pressures, it is difficult to achieve oxygen saturations above 90%. List four potentially reversal causes for this.

2 marks
(0.5 mark for each correct stem)

- Pneumothorax.
- Lung collapse.
- Severe bronchospasm.
- Pulmonary embolism.

5) Pulmonary embolism is suspected, but is subsequently excluded by a negative CT pulmonary angiogram. A maximal PEEP at 20cmH$_2$O with inverse ratio ventilation and varying tidal volumes are tried with no significant improvement in oxygen saturations. Prone position ventilation is considered. How is prone positioning meant to improve oxygenation?

3 marks
(0.5 mark for each correct stem, with a maximum of 3 marks)

Prone positioning has been used in mechanically ventilated patients with severe ARDS. The prone position is believed to improve oxygenation and gas exchange through a number of postulated mechanisms. These include:

- Improved ventilation-perfusion matching by preferentially ventilating previously dependent areas.
- Redistribution of oedema with improved drainage of secretions.

- Physical weight redistribution of the mediastinal structures onto the sternum away from the dependent areas.
- Increase in functional residual capacity (FRC).
- Reduced atelectasis.
- The gravitational theory:
  - gravity displacing the heart with a decreased amount of lung compression;
  - unhindered diaphragmatic function.

6) A referral to the nearest centre offering extracorporeal membrane oxygenation (ECMO) is made. What types of ECMO are there and what is the most likely type this patient will benefit from?

1 mark

- Veno-venous.
- Veno-arterial.
- This patient will benefit from veno-venous ECMO.

7) Explain the principles of veno-venous ECMO and how this may help the patient in particular.

4 marks
(1 mark for each correct stem, with a maximum of 4 marks)

- Large cannulae (16-22Fr gauge) placed in a large central vein act to drain blood.
- With veno-venous ECMO, bicaval cannulae are often used.
- Blood flows through a circuit with tubing.
- Blood passes through a membrane oxygenator and heat exchanger.
- A pump can be incorporated.
- The oxygenated blood is returned to the venous circulation distal to the initial drainage site.

8) This patient does not have cardiogenic dysfunction. Veno-venous ECMO is beneficial for patients with severe respiratory pathology resistant to conventional ventilator measures. List four complications with ECMO.

2 marks (0.5 mark for each correct stem, with a maximum of 2 marks)

- Bleeding.
- Haemolysis.
- Equipment failure — oxygenator, pump, circuit failure.
- Clot formation — hence anticoagulation is required.
- Air embolism.

Top Tip

In 2013, Guérin *et al* carried out a randomised controlled trial — the PROSEVA trial — in which 466 patients were randomised to either a group receiving prone position sessions or supine position care [1]. The study looked to ascertain if early proning for 16 hours a session in moderate to severe ARDS would improve 28-day mortality. The results found a 28-day mortality of 16% in the prone group compared with a mortality of 32.8% in the supine group (p<0.0001).

References

1.   Guérin C, Reignier J, Richard J-C, *et al*. Prone positioning in severe acute respiratory distress syndrome. *N Engl J Med* 2013; 368: 2159-68.

Panton-Valentine leukocidin (PVL) pneumonia and antibiotics

You are the doctor on duty for the ICU and have been asked to review a 47-year-old man who has walked into the emergency department complaining of a cough for the last 3 days. Over the past 24 hours he has found that his breathing has become progressively more difficult.

On your arrival he is saturating at 98% on 15L of oxygen via a non-rebreathe mask with a respiratory rate of 30 breaths per minute. You notice that his temperature is 39.5°C, he is tachycardic and his blood pressure is 98/45mmHg.

1) The emergency department nurse hands you his arterial blood gas (ABG) (Table 3.6). Please summarise the ABG.

1 mark

Table 3.6. Arterial blood gas results.	
pH	7.23
PaO_2	8.4kPa
$PaCO_2$	3.2kPa
HCO_3^-	23mmol/L
Lactate	6.9mmol/L
BE	-11mmol/L

- Metabolic acidosis with attempted respiratory compensation.

2) What further tests would you perform?

Blood tests:

- Full blood count.
- Urea and electrolytes.
- Liver biochemistry.
- C-reactive protein (CRP).
- Blood culture.

Other tests:

- *Legionella* and pneumococcal urinary antigens.
- Urine dipstick.
- Sputum culture.
- Chest X-ray.
- Electrocardiogram.

4 marks

(0.5 mark for each correct stem, with a maximum of 4 marks)

3) A chest X-ray is performed (● Figure 3.6). Please outline any abnormality.

- There is an opacification in the right middle lobe and lower lobe.

1 mark

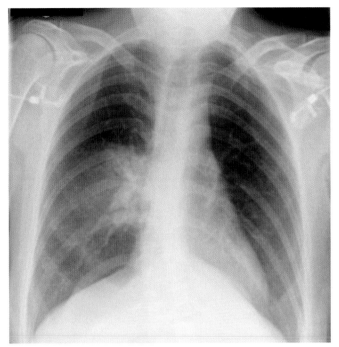

Figure 3.6.

4) What is the most likely diagnosis?   1 mark

- Infection. This could be bacterial, viral or fungal (though less likely).

5) What are the likely micro-organisms causing this infection?   2 marks

This case history and presentation is suspicious of a community-acquired pneumonia (CAP). The commonest pathogens for a CAP are:

- *Streptococcus pneumoniae.*

- *Haemophilus influenzae.*
- *Moraxella catarrhalis.*

6) What antibiotic regime would you use to treat this patient?   2 marks

- Adhere to local policy to account for bacterial resistance patterns.
- Common organisms as well as atypical organisms should be covered in the first instance.
  - penicillin or cephalosporin; *plus*
  - macrolide (for atypical cover), e.g. benzylpenicillin plus clarithromycin.

7) Why don't penicillins work against atypical pneumonia?   2 marks

- Penicillins act on bacterial cell wall synthesis.
- Many atypical organisms such as *Mycoplasma* and *Chlamydia* do not have accessible cell walls.
- Therefore, penicillins don't work.

8) How do macrolides work?   2 marks

Macrolides:

- Are bacteriostatic.
- Act on RNA-dependent protein synthesis.

9) The patient is admitted to the ICU and on the following day he is still noted to be febrile; he   2 marks
(0.5 mark for each correct stem)

deteriorates and requires intubation. On closed suctioning, blood-stained sputum is noted. The on-call microbiologist calls stating that there are Gram-positive cocci in his blood culture.

The patient's morning blood test results are shown below (● Table 3.7). Summarise the results and suggest a likely cause.

Table 3.7. Blood test results.	
Hb	107g/L
WCC	2.1×10^9/L
Platelets	120×10^9/L
Neutrophils	1.5×10^9/L
Na$^+$	135mmol/L
K$^+$	4.6mmol/L
Urea	8.9mmol/L
Creatinine	120μmol/L
CRP	450mg/L
CK	750ng/L

There is:

- Leukopaenia.
- Raised C-reactive protein (CRP).
- Raised creatine kinase (CK).
- The most likely cause is a PVL *Staphylococcus aureus* pneumonia.

10) He is diagnosed with a PVL *Staphylococcus* necrotising pneumonia. How would your treatment change?

1 mark
(1 mark for IVIg)

- Continue supportive treatment and modify antibiotics.
- Current guidelines suggest treatment with intravenous immunoglobulins (IVIg).

11) What antibiotics would you consider to treat a PVL necrotising pneumonia and would they work in this case?

2 marks

- Clindamycin or linezolid (decreases toxin production); used along with rifampicin (staphylococcal clearance).

Top Tip

The British Thoracic Society has produced a quick reference on CAP. The section on atypical CAP is important to understand. The guidance states the following on PVL pneumonia [1]:

"Specific issues regarding Panton-Valentine leukocidin-producing *Staphylococcus aureus* (PVL-SA).

- PVL-SA infection is a rare cause of high severity pneumonia, and can be associated with rapid lung cavitation and multiorgan failure. Such patients should be considered for critical care admission.

- If PVL-SA necrotising pneumonia is strongly suspected or confirmed, clinicians should liaise urgently with microbiology in relation to further antibiotic management, and consider referral to the respiratory medicine department for clinical management advice.

- Current recommendations for the antibiotic management of strongly suspected necrotising pneumonia include the addition of a combination of intravenous linezolid 600mg twice daily, intravenous clindamycin 1.2g four times a day and intravenous rifampicin 600mg twice daily to the initial empirical antibiotic regimen. As soon as PVL-SA infection is either confirmed or excluded, antibiotic therapy should be narrowed accordingly."

References

1. Lim WS, Baudouin SV, George RC, *et al.* BTS guidelines for the management of community-acquired pneumonia in adults: update 2009. *Thorax* 2009; 64(Suppl 3): iii1-55.

Renal replacement therapy

This station will have questions on renal replacement therapy.

1) What types of renal replacement therapy (RRT) are commonly available on ICU?

1 mark
(all 3 should be listed to gain 1 mark)

- Continuous veno-venous haemofiltration (CVVHF).
- Continuous veno-venous diafiltration (CVVDF).
- Continuous veno-venous haemodiafiltration (CVVHDF).

2) What are the functional principles behind RRT?

1 mark
(0.5 mark for each correct stem)

- Haemofiltration — convection or solvent drag.
- Dialysis — diffusion.

3) You are presented with the following diagram overleaf (● Figure 3.7). Label the schematic diagram.

3 marks
(0.5 mark for each correct stem)

- A — replacement fluid.
- B — arterial limb of vascath from patient.
- C — venous limb of vascath to patient.
- D — haemofilter.
- E — pump taking filtrate away from patient.
- F — pump bringing dialysate to the patient.

CVVHDF

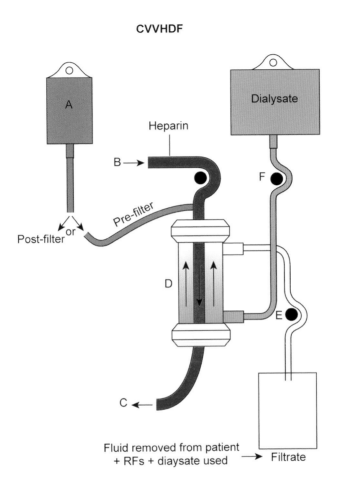

Figure 3.7.

4) List the indications for RRT.

3 marks

(0.5 mark for each correct stem)

- Symptomatic uraemia, for example, pericarditis, encephalopathy.
- Renal failure with associated metabolic acidosis.

- Hyperkalaemia.
- Fluid overload (secondary to heart failure, renal failure or hepatic failure).
- Temperature control — to induce hypothermia.
- Drug and toxin removal, for example, lithium, salicylates.

5) **What variables would you need to prescribe when commencing RRT? Please give examples of a standard prescription for each.**

4 marks
(1 mark for each correct stem and correct prescription example)

- Rate of filtration at 25-30ml/kg/hr.
- Rate at which blood is drawn from the patient — 250-300ml/min.
- Fluid balance aim — for example, negative 1L over a 24-hour period or neutral balance at 24 hours.
- Anticoagulation prescription, for example, with unfractionated heparin.

6) **What are the options for anticoagulation?**

3 marks
(0.5 mark for each correct stem, with a maximum of 3 marks)

- Systemic unfractionated IV heparin.
- Heparinisation of the RRT equipment alone.
- Low-molecular-weight heparin.
- Prostacycline.
- Citrate and calcium.
- Factor Xa Inhibitor — fondaparinux (either answer sufficient for the mark).
- Direct thrombin inhibitor — bivalirudin.

7) What scoring system are you aware of to grade heparin-induced thrombotic thrombocytopenic syndrome (HITTS)?

1 mark

(the 4Ts system and each constituent must be listed correctly for the full mark, otherwise no marks will be given)

A system that grades 4Ts:

- Severity of **T**hrombocytopenia.
- **T**iming of platelet decrease.
- **T**hrombosis.
- Can the **T**hrombocytopenia be due to any other reason?

8) What types of HITTS are there?

1 mark

(0.5 mark for each correct stem)

- Type I — non-immune, less severe condition.
- Type II — immune-mediated.

9) What is the management of suspected HITTS?

- Stop heparin.

0.5 mark

- Avoid platelet transfusion — as this can worsen the thrombocytopenia.

0.5 mark

- The patient is in a pro-thrombotic state and requires urgent alternative anticoagulation.

1 mark

- Diagnosis is through:

1 mark

  - clinical suspicion;
  - high 4Ts system score;
  - laboratory tests:
    - antigen assays are quick but not high in sensitivity and specificity;
    - functional assays, whilst having a high specificity, are expensive and take a lot of time.

References

1.   Scott I, Webster NR. Heparin-induced thrombocytopenia: is there
      a role for direct thrombin inhibitors in therapy? *J Intensive Care
      Soc* 2014; 15(2): 131-4.

Electrocardiography — set 3

1) This is an electrocardiogram (ECG) of a 68-year-old man who has a history of hypertension, diabetes, an expansive smoking history and marked obesity (Figure 3.8). Please describe this ECG.

3 marks
(0.5 mark for each correct stem, with a maximum of 3 marks)

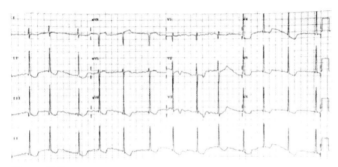

Figure 3.8.

- Rate — variable rate between 75-90.
- Rhythm — irregularly irregular.
- Axis — normal axis.
- P-wave morphology and P-R interval — P-waves are not clearly and consistently seen, hence the P-R interval is uninterpretable.
- QRS complex — normal QRS complex.
- ST segments — ST depression in V4, V5, V6 II, III and aVF.
- T-wave morphology — T-wave inversion V2-V3.
- Other overall comments — evidence of global myocardial ischaemia in the inferolateral leads.

2) What is the diagnosis?   1 mark

- Inferolateral myocardial ischaemia, with atrial fibrillation.

3) How would you manage this patient if they had ongoing chest pain and were cardiovascularly unstable?   4 marks

- Acute assessment, resuscitation and management should be undertaken to follow an 'airway, breathing, circulation, disability and exposure' approach.
- The patient will require institution of acute coronary syndrome management; however, concurrent urgent referral for cardiology advice should be sought.
- Referral for an urgent cardiology review as this patient may:
  - require expedited angiography;
  - institution of additional pharmacological agents such as:
    - a glycoprotein IIb/IIIa inhibitor infusion, for example, a tirofiban infusion;
    - a glyceryl trinitrate (GTN) infusion;
    - a newer ADP P2Y12 receptor blocker, such as prasugrel or ticagrelor, may be requested above clopidogrel;
    - an alternative to low-molecular-weight heparin, such as fondaparinux.

4) This ECG belongs to an 82-year-old male with known cerebrovascular disease who has presented with palpitations (● Figure 3.9). Please describe this ECG.

3 marks
(0.5 mark for each correct stem, with a maximum of 3 marks)

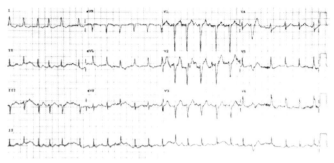

Figure 3.9.

- Rate — due to the irregular rhythm the ventricular rate is between 100-140 beats per minute.
- Rhythm — irregularly irregular rhythm.
- Axis — normal axis.
- P-wave morphology and P-R interval — P-waves are not clearly and consistently seen, hence the P-R interval is uninterpretable.
- QRS complex — normal QRS complex.
- ST segments — isoelectric.
- T-wave morphology — normal T-waves.

5) What is the diagnosis?   1 mark

- Atrial fibrillation (AF).

6) What would be your management strategy if   2 marks
this patient with newly diagnosed atrial
fibrillation is cardiovascularly compromised?

- Acute assessment, resuscitation and management should be undertaken to follow an 'airway, breathing, circulation, disability and exposure' approach.

- This patient has newly diagnosed AF and is cardiovascularly compromised, and as such the patient requires electrical cardioversion.

7) This ECG belongs to a 62-year-old man (● Figure 3.10). Please describe this ECG.

3 marks
(0.5 mark for each correct stem, with a maximum of 3 marks)

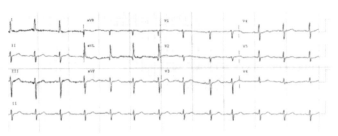

Figure 3.10.

- Rate — 75 bpm.
- Rhythm — sinus rhythm (SR).
- Axis — right axis deviation.
- P-wave morphology and P-R interval — abnormal P-wave morphology — P-mitrale.
- QRS complex — normal QRS complex.
- ST segments — normal.
- T-wave morphology — normal T-waves.

8) What is the diagnosis?

1 mark

- P-mitrale.

9) What is the cause of this main abnormality? 2 marks

- Left atrial enlargement with the commonest causes secondary to:
  - mitral valve disease — usually insufficiency;
  - congestive cardiac failure.

References

1. Biondi-Zoccai G, Lotrionte M, Gaita F. Alternatives to clopidogrel for acute coronary syndromes: prasugrel or ticagrelor? *World J Cardiol* 2010; 2(6): 131.

Radiology — set 3

1) The following CT scan was obtained from a 67-year-old female who was involved in a road traffic accident (● Figure 3.11). What does this CT scan show?

3 marks

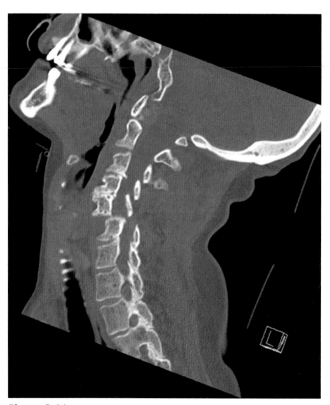

Figure 3.11.

- Anterior slip of C5 on C6.
- Dislocation of the left C5-C6 facet joints.
- Narrowing of the spinal cord.

2) How would you manage this injury?   3 marks

● This patient has an unstable C-spine.
● Collar and blocks, manual in-line stabilisation and log rolling if necessary.
● Discussion with orthopaedics/neurosurgeons.

3) The following chest X-ray was obtained from an 85-year-old patient (● Figure 3.12). What is the abnormality?   1 mark

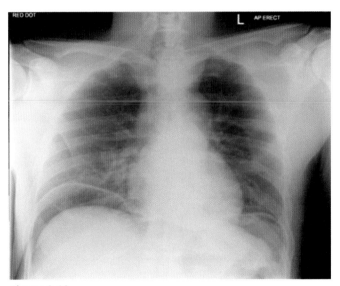

Figure 3.12.

● Free air under both sides of the diaphragm.

4) List the causes of this condition.   3 marks

(for 3 correct

- Bowel perforation, e.g. duodenal/gastric ulcer   stems)
  perforation.
- Malignancy.
- Iatrogenic, e.g. post-laparoscopy.
- Penetrating trauma.
- Necrotising bowel infection.

5) The following X-ray was obtained from a 25-   2 marks
   year-old male who was brought into the
   emergency department following a traumatic
   injury (● Figure 3.13). What abnormalities
   are present on this X-ray?

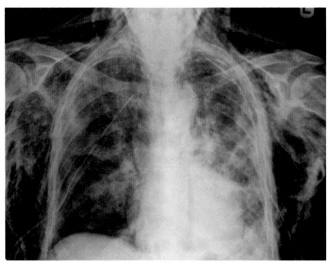

Figure 3.13.

- Massive subcutaneous emphysema.
- Bilateral intercostal drains.

6) What complication could this cause?   1 mark

- Restriction of chest wall movement leading to impaired respiratory mechanics and difficulty with ventilation.

7) How would you treat this complication?   1 mark

- Referral to surgeons for consideration of fasciotomies.

8) The following chest X-ray was taken of a 30-year-old male who presented with acute shortness of breath and pleuritic chest pain (● Figure 3.14). What abnormality is present?   1 mark

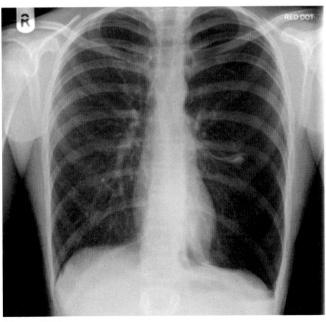

Figure 3.14.

- Large left-sided pneumothorax.

9) How would you manage this patient? 2 marks

- If there are signs of tension, then needle decompression is required.
- Placement of an intercostal drain, connected to an underwater seal.

10) What are the risk factors for spontaneous pneumothorax? 3 marks

(0.5 mark for each correct stem)

- Male.
- Smoking.
- Age (20-40 years).
- Underlying lung disease.
- Past history of pneumothoraces.
- Mechanical ventilation.

Chapter 4

Rhabdomyolysis

A 22-year-old man undertook a 15-mile charity run. The man's partner had revealed that he had not prepared well having never undertaken any training runs.

He has been brought to the emergency department having collapsed towards the end of the event. He has severe leg cramps and back pain and weakness in the legs.

1) The patient has the following blood results (●) Table 4.1) and an arterial blood gas (ABG)(●) 2 marks
(0.5 mark for each correct stem)

Table 4.1. Blood test results.	
Hb	141g/L
WCC	11.3×10^9/L
Platelets	347×10^9/L
MCV	89fL
RBC	5.4×10^{12}/L
MCH	29pg
MCHC	324g/L
	Continued

Table 4.1. Blood test results *continued*.

Na$^+$	143mmol/L
K$^+$	6.0mmol/L
Urea	13.6mmol/L
Creatinine	96μmol/L
CRP	84mg/L
CK	22,000i.u./L

Table 4.2. Arterial blood gas results.

pH	7.23
PO$_2$	10.5kPa
PCO$_2$	3.3kPa
HCO$_3^-$	17.3mmol/L
Cl$^-$	87mmol/L
Lactate	4.5mmol/L
BE	-6.5mmol/L

Table 4.2). Summarise and comment on these results.

- Hyperkalaemia.
- Significantly raised creatine kinase (CK).
- Metabolic acidosis.
- Raised lactate.

2) Based on the information what is the most likely diagnosis?

1 mark

(0.5 mark for each correct stem)

- Rhabdomyolysis (exercise-induced).

- Potential heat injury.

(If the candidate fails to correctly diagnose, please inform them "You have diagnosed rhabdomyolysis".)

3) List four other causes of rhabdomyolysis.

4 marks

(1 mark for each correct stem, with a maximum of 4 marks)

- Trauma — burns, crush injuries, associated compartment syndrome.
- Prolonged immobility.
- Drugs — statins, cocaine, amphetamines.
- Malignant hyperpyrexia.
- Serotonin syndrome.
- Neuroleptic malignant syndrome.
- Metabolic emergencies — phaeochromocytoma or thyroid storm.

4) Please describe the pathophysiology of rhabdomyolysis.

5 marks

- The underlying precipitant cause as from the list above, be it traumatic or non-traumatic causes the calcium-ATPase pump on the myocytes to be damaged and fail.
- There is a subsequent increase in sarcoplasmic calcium causing unopposed contraction.
- This activates intracellular proteases.
- This leads to skeletal muscle disintegration.
- Release of intracellular proteins and electrolytes into the circulation.

5) List the biochemical changes that may be seen in addition to the changes seen above.

2 marks
(1 mark for each correct stem)

- Increase in plasma phosphate, uric acid, myoglobin.
- Decrease in plasma calcium.

6) List the major associated complications.

2 marks
(1 mark for each correct stem — must include AKI, with a maximum of 2 marks)

- Acute kidney injury (AKI).
- Electrolyte emergencies:
  - hyperkalaemia;
  - hyperphosphataemia;
  - hypocalcaemia.
- Disseminated intravascular coagulopathy.

7) What other investigations would you order for this patient and why?

1.5 marks
(0.5 mark for each correct stem)

Bedside:

- ECG — changes associated with hyperkalaemia.

Laboratory:

- Coagulation profile — due to potential disseminated intravascular coagulation (DIC).
- Myoglobin levels (urinary levels) — characteristic marker of rhabdomyolysis and AKI.

8) Please review this ECG (● Figure 4.1) and present the key salient features.

2.5 marks
(0.5 mark for each correct stem, with a maximum of 2.5 marks)

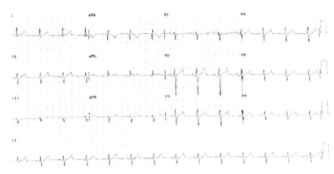

Figure 4.1.

- Sinus rhythm, rate of between 90-100 beats per minute.
- Left axis deviation.
- PR interval 0.24 seconds — 1st degree heart block.
- QRS complex of normal duration.
- T-waves appear peaked in V2 and V3.

Top Tip

This OSCE has focused on the AKI associated with rhabdomyolysis. The pathophysiology associated with the AKI is related to:

- Renal tubular — obstruction, injury and ischaemia.
- There is a sudden profound burden of myoglobin on the renal tubules.

- The myoglobin interacts with proteins forming brown granular casts, therefore causing tubular obstruction.
- The acidic conditions promote further cast formation.
- Myoglobin also inhibits endogenous nitric oxide; hence, there is unopposed renal vasoconstriction which leads to renal ischaemia.

The other area to be proficiently familiar with is the management of AKI in the context of rhabdomyolysis.

Specific management:

- Fluid resuscitate to achieve a urine output of >3ml/kg or 300ml/hr.
- Sodium bicarbonate 50-100mmol boluses targeting a urine pH >6.5.
- Mannitol may flush out nephrotoxic agents and act as a free radical scavenger.

For the management of associated hyperkalaemia, see the ECG OSCE in Chapter 2 on hyperkalaemia.

References

1.   Bosch X, Poch E, Grau JM. Rhabdomyolysis and acute kidney injury. *N Engl J Med* 2009; 361: 62-72.

Professionalism — NG tube in the lung

You are the senior doctor on the ICU and have been asked to discuss a case with one of your colleagues who is quite junior.

The patient had a nasogastric (NG) tube inserted by this doctor yesterday evening, a chest X-ray was not performed before feeding was commenced and overnight the patient has deteriorated. A subsequent X-ray has shown that the NG tube was placed in the lung and there is extensive evidence of nasogastric feed within the left lung field.

You have been asked to discuss this case with the doctor involved.

In this scenario the junior doctor will be played by an actor.

1) Please discuss the case with the junior colleague and outline the first step with regard to this incident.

The candidate:

• Provides an appropriate introduction, including their name, role and the reason for the discussion.	1 mark
• Checks that the doctor is comfortable to have a discussion at this time.	1 mark
• Checks that they do not want anyone else present.	1 mark
• Allows the doctor to explain the circumstances surrounding the incident, without unnecessary interruption.	2 marks

2) The doctor will explain that it was a busy shift,   2 marks
    that the NG tube went in easily, the patient did
    not cough and that they performed the
    'Whoosh test'. As everything seemed OK and
    the radiographer was busy in the emergency
    department, they thought that feeding was
    more important.

The candidate:

● Explains what has happened and checks that the
  doctor understands the seriousness of the incident.

3) The junior colleague will imply that this is "just
    one of those things" and "nothing to get too
    worried about".

The candidate:

● Explains that this incident is a 'never event' and as   1 mark
  such must be reported via the hospital's reporting
  system.
● Advises that an incident form will be completed and   1 mark
  the event will be investigated.
● Stresses that the purpose of any investigation is to   1 mark
  identify failings in the system/training rather than to
  apportion blame.

4) The junior doctor will suggest that an incident   1 mark
    form is not filled in and asks you to "keep this
    between us".

The candidate:

- Again states that an incident form must be filled in.

5) If not already covered by the candidate, the junior doctor will ask "what happens next?"

The candidate:

• States that the family of the patient will be informed of the incident.	1 mark
• Explains that an investigation of the circumstances will be carried out, and a report will be prepared and fed back to all parties involved.	1 mark
• Advises that the junior doctor will need to declare this incident on their revalidation documents.	1 mark
• Offers sources of support for the junior doctor, e.g. education supervisor, defence union, hospital support unit.	1 mark
• Ensures that the junior doctor is fit to continue working.	1 mark
• Suggests an interim action plan to prevent such incidents occurring again, such as making sure a senior colleague checks any NG tube placement, arranging for further instruction on NG tube insertion.	2 marks
• Speaks clearly in a non-judgemental way, checks the junior doctor's understanding and allows for questions.	2 marks

References

1. National Patient Safety Agency. Patient Safety Alert NPSA/2011/PSA002: Reducing the harm caused by misplaced nasogastric feeding tubes in adults, children and infants. National Patient Saftey Agency, March 2011. http://www.nrls.npsa.nhs.uk/EasySiteWeb/getresource.axd?AssetID=129697&.

Acute pancreatitis

A 71-year-old gentleman with known gallstone disease presents to the emergency department with abdominal pain. The patient has a history of ischaemic heart disease which resulted in a non-ST-segment elevation myocardial infarction (NSTEMI) requiring management with percutaneous coronary intervention with stent placement 1 month ago. The patient had been started on oral clopidogrel. The cholecystectomy planned for gallstone disease was postponed under the recommendation of the cardiology team who had requested the clopidogrel be ideally continued for a minimum of 6 weeks. Other medical history includes obstructive sleep apnoea (OSA).

The emergency department physician has asked for an intensive care review.

1) Upon arrival you are presented with the following blood gas results (● Table 4.3). Please summarise the results.

2 marks
(1 mark for summary and 1 mark for explanation)

Table 4.3. Arterial blood gas results.

FiO$_2$	0.21
pH	7.33
PaO$_2$	7.89kPa
PaCO$_2$	7.9kPa
HCO$_3^-$	34.5mmol/L
BE	5.3mmol/L

- There is a chronic respiratory acidosis, indicated by the raised HCO_3^- and BE.
- This may be due to the patient's history of OSA.

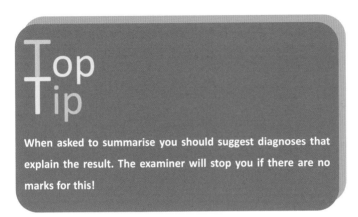

Top Tip

When asked to summarise you should suggest diagnoses that explain the result. The examiner will stop you if there are no marks for this!

2) The emergency department team presents you with further history; the patient presents with acute abdominal pain. The following blood test results have been obtained (● Table 4.4). Further biochemical tests including calcium, LDH, and liver biochemistry reveal the calcium to be 2.15mmol/L, with a normal

1 mark

Table 4.4. Blood test results.	
WCC	15.7×10^9/L
Urea	9.3mmol/L
Creatinine	147µmol/L
Serum lipase	6000i.u./L

LDH but a raised ALT of 201mmol/L. What is the most likely diagnosis?

- Acute pancreatitis.

3) Prior to admission, the emergency department team asks you to calculate the Glasgow score for this patient and explain to the assembled medical students how this score is used to guide critical care admission.

2 marks
(1 mark for the calculation and 1 mark for appropriate interpretation)

(The candidate will be given the Glasgow score template to calculate it — see the Top Tip on p196!)

- Age — age >55 years = 1.
- Partial pressure of arterial oxygen — PaO_2 <8kPa = 1.
- White cell count — WCC >15 x 10^9/L= 1.
- Serum calcium — Ca ≥2.00mmol/L = 0.
- Serum urea — urea ≤16mmol/L = 0.
- Enzymes lactate dehydrogenase and AST or ALT — if LDH >600i.u./L or AST/ALT >200i.u./L score = 1.
- Serum albumin — alb <32g/L = 1 and alb ≥32g/L = 0.
- Glucose — glucose ≤ x 10mmol/L = 0.

The Glasgow score is 4. A score of 3 or more indicates that a critical care referral for at least high dependency care is required.

4) You clinically suspect acute gallstone pancreatitis. What is the pathophysiology of this?

2 marks
(0.5 mark for each correct stem)

- Acute pancreatitis is a condition spanning from mild symptomology through to severe forms resulting in acute necrotising pancreatitis.

- It is a condition where a trigger has resulted in the proteolytic enzymes of the pancreas such as trypsin to be activated and proceed to autodigest the pancreatic parenchyma.
- This may result in haemorrhagic necrosis.
- The disease process can trigger a systemic inflammatory response with multi-organ failure.

5) List the commonest causes of acute pancreatitis.

2 marks
(0.5 mark for each correct stem, with a maximum of 2 marks)

- Gallstones.
- Alcohol.
- Other causes include trauma, viral causes such as Ebstein-Barr virus (EBV) or *Cytomegalovirus* (CMV), autoimmune diseases such as systemic lupus erythematosus (SLE), scorpion stings, drugs such as sulphasalazine, azathioprine, NSAIDs with metronidazole, sodium valproate or tetracyclines.

6) What other investigations would you consider in gallstone pancreatitis?

2 marks
(0.5 mark for each correct stem, with a maximum of 2 marks)

- Abdominal ultrasound.
- Contrast-enhanced CT.
- MRI.
- Magnetic resonance cholangiopancreatography (MRCP).
- Endoscopic retrograde cholangiopancreatography (ERCP) for stone removal.

7) List some other scoring systems associated with acute pancreatitis.

2 marks
(1 mark for each correct stem)

- Ranson's score — see the Top Tip on p197.
- CT-guided scoring systems such as the Balthazar CT Severity Index.

8) What are the Atlanta Criteria 2013?

2 marks
(1 mark for what it is and another mark for the mild, moderate and severe classification)

- An international consensus was sought in classifying acute pancreatitis.

The classification is as follows:

- Mild acute pancreatitis — the most common form, has no organ failure, local or systemic complications and usually resolves in the first week.
- Moderately severe acute pancreatitis — is defined by the presence of transient organ failure, local complications or exacerbation of comorbid disease.
- Severe acute pancreatitis — is defined by persistent organ failure, that is, organ failure >48h. Local complications are peripancreatic fluid collections, pancreatic and peripancreatic necrosis (sterile or infected), pseudocysts and walled-off necrosis (sterile or infected).

9) How would you manage a patient with gallstone pancreatitis?

5 marks
(1 mark for each correctly explained stem, with a maximum of 5 marks)

- Acute assessment, resuscitation and management should be undertaken to follow an 'airway, breathing, circulation, disability and exposure' approach.

- Appreciate that the patient could develop SIRS and multi-organ failure.
- Involve colleagues — gastroenterologists and general surgeons.
- It is unlikely that the patient will have an emergency cholecystectomy whilst there is an acutely inflamed pancreas.
- However, MRCP and ERCP are important early options.
- Early enteral feeding.
- Antibiotics are not part of standard treatment unless there is evidence of an infection — either a pancreatic abscess, or collections.
- The role of surgery is very limited and reserved for:
  - radiological-guided drainage of abscesses, cysts or pseudocysts;
  - in severe cases where acute pancreatitis causes abdominal compartment syndrome, hence requiring decompressive laparostomy.

References

1. Shanbhogue AKP, Fasih N, Surabhi VR, *et al*. A clinical and radiologic review of uncommon types and causes of pancreatitis. *Radiographics* 2009; 29(4): 1003-26.

2. Banks PA, Freeman ML, Fass R, *et al*. Practice guidelines in acute pancreatitis. *Am J Gastroenterol* 2006; 101(10): 2379-400.

3. Corfield AP, Williamson RCN, McMahon MJ, *et al*. Prediction of severity in acute pancreatitis: prospective comparison of three prognostic indices. *Lancet* 1985; 24: 403-7.

4. Ranson JHC, Rifkind KM, Roses DF, *et al*. Prognostic signs and the role of operative management in acute pancreatitis. *Surg Gynecol Obstet* 1974; 139: 69-81.

5. Chatzicostas C, Roussomoustakaki M, Vardas E, *et al*. Balthazar computed tomography severity index is superior to Ranson criteria and APACHE II and III scoring systems in predicting acute pancreatitis outcome. *J Clin Gastroenterol* 2003; 36(3): 253-60.

Top Tip

The Glasgow scoring system was implemented in the case described above. The factors used are:

- Age:

  Age >55 years = 1 and age $\leq$55 years = 0.
- Partial pressure of arterial oxygen:

  PaO_2 <8kPa = 1 and PaO_2 >= 8kPa = 0.
- White cell count:

  WCC >15 x 10^9/L= 1 and WCC $\leq$15 x 10^9/L = 0.
- Serum calcium:

  Ca <2.00mmo/L = 1 and Ca $\geq$2.00mmol/L = 0.
- Serum urea:

  Urea >16mmol/L = 1 and urea $\leq$16mmol/L = 0.
- Enzymes lactate dehydrogenase and AST or ALT:

  If LDH >600i.u./L or AST/ALT >200i.u./L score = 1.

  LDH $\leq$600i.u./L or AST/ALT $\leq$200i.u./L score = 0.
- Serum albumin:

  Alb <32g/L = 1 and Alb $\geq$32g/L = 0.
- Glucose:

  Glucose >10mmo/L = 1 and glucose $\leq$ x 10mmol/L = 0.

A score of >3 indicates acute severe pancreatitis. A score of <3 indicates acute mild pancreatitis. It was suggested that a score of 3 or more should be referred for critical care in the HDU or ICU.

Top Tip

The Ranson criteria look at the following:

At 0 hours:

- Age — >55 years.
- WCC — >16 x 10^9/L.
- Blood glucose — 11.1mmol/L.
- LDH — >350i.u./L.
- AST — >250i.u./L.

At 48 hours:

- Haematocrit — fall by >10%.
- Blood urea nitrogen — increase by >5mg/dL.
- Serum calcium — <2mmol/L.
- PaO_2 — <8kPa.

The presence of one to three of these criteria represents mild pancreatitis. The mortality rate rises significantly with four or more criteria.

6.   Banks PA, Bollen TL, Dervenis C, *et al*. Classification of acute pancreatitis - 2012: revision of the Atlanta classification and definitions by international consensus. *Gut* 2013; 62(1): 102-11.

Pulmonary infiltrates

You are called to the emergency department to review a 30-year-old patient who is 32 weeks' pregnant. She has presented with a 3-day history of dry cough and now is feeling short of breath.

She has a heart rate of 110 beats per minute, which is irregular with a blood pressure of 110/70mmHg and a respiratory rate of 27 breaths per minute.

1) What investigations would you order for this patient?

1 mark

(all 3 stems must be listed)

- Chest X-ray.
- Echocardiography.
- ECG.

2) You are presented with the following chest X-ray (● Figure 4.2). Please describe any abnormal features.

1 mark

- There is bilateral shadowing across both lung fields.
- This is suggestive of pulmonary oedema.

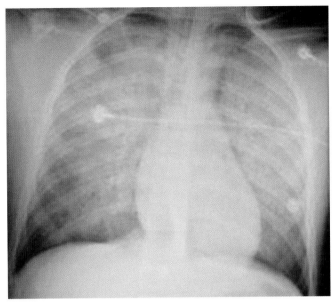

Figure 4.2.

3)   What are your differential diagnoses?

4 marks
(1 mark for
each correct
stem and sub-
stem)

- Pulmonary oedema:
    - cardiogenic;
    - valve disease — congential or acquired;
    - iatrogenic fluid overload;
    - renal failure;
    - liver failure.
- Infection:
    - bacterial, viral, fungal or protozoal (though unlikely).
- Autoimmune:
    - Goodpasture's syndrome, pulmonary fibrosis.
- Acute respiratory distress syndrome (ARDS).

4) How would you manage this patient?

5 marks

(1 mark for each correct stem, with a maximum of 5 marks)

The following measures would form the basis of management:

- Acute assessment, resuscitation and management should be undertaken to follow an 'airway, breathing, circulation, disability and exposure' approach.
- A multi-disciplinary approach.
- Beta-blocker for rate control.
- Consider a diuretic management.
- Consider intubation. If intubation is required then anaesthetic assistance will be required and plans for a rapid sequence induction (RSI) should be made.
- Delivery of the baby.

Top Tip

If any procedure is mentioned, for example, intubation, then it is important to factor in the repercussions of the preparation required. All procedures should follow a 'preparation, preparation and preparation strategy' in a swift and timely manner. To elaborate this is:

- Preparation of the patient: consent, positioning, administration of additional drugs, for example, antacids, sodium citrate and stopping the nasogastric feeding.

- Preparation of the personnel and environment: anaesthetic nurse, additional staff for mobilising the difficult airway trolley, personnel to help with the application of cricoid pressure and correct named identified personnel to help with a difficult intubation.

- Preparation of equipment and drugs: in this example drugs for an RSI along with emergency drugs correctly drawn up, labelled and made ready (propofol, rocuronium, opiate, metaraminol, atropine, ephedrine, adrenaline, intravenous fluids, saline flushes). Equipment may include mobilising, and also checking, the intubation kit including laryngoscopes, gum elastic bougie and end-tidal carbon dioxide monitoring as well as the difficult airway trolley.

- It is now good practice as identified from the National Audit Project 4 (NAP4) that a moment to pause and challenge the airway operator as to the necessary preparation, along with a declaration to the team regarding the airway strategy and plan, should be done just before intubation.

In an OSCE question based on any procedure, an early declaration to the examiner that you will take time to prepare the patient, personnel, environment and the necessary equipment and drugs, allows you to score marks and to organise your thoughts around this framework. Thus, it is harder to miss important facts, which could score you that valuable extra mark to pass the exam! Hence, preparation, preparation and preparation.

5) The obstetricians deliver the baby. However, she fails to improve and an echocardiogram diagnoses mitral stenosis. What is the most common cause of mitral stenosis in pregnancy?

1 mark

- Rheumatic fever.

6) How would you manage the patient?

4 marks

(1 mark for each correct stem, with a maximum of 4 marks)

- Beta-blockers.
- Diuretics.
- Percutaneous mitral valvuloplasty.
- Valve replacement.
- Anticoagulation — these patients have a high risk of thromboembolic disease.

7) You refer her to the cardiothoracic surgeons. What are the salient equipment features of this chest radiograph (● Figure 4.3) and what does this indicate with regard to what has happened to the patient?

4 marks

(1 mark for each correct stem, with a maximum of 4 marks)

This is a supine portable chest radiograph. There is:

- A correctly sited nasogastric tube.
- A correctly sited endotracheal tube.
- A correctly placed left internal jugular central line.
- A mitral valve replacement.
- A large catheter on the right side indicating the patient is being supported with extracorporeal membrane oxygenation.

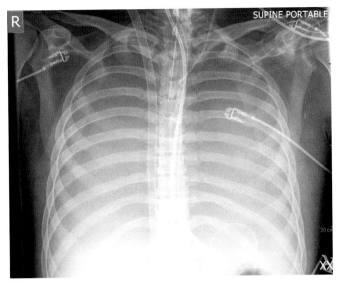

Figure 4.3.

References

1. Burt CC, Durbridge J. Management of cardiac disease in pregnancy. *Cont Educ Anaesth Crit Care Pain* 2009; 9(2): 44-7.

Septic shock and fluids

A 24-year-old man has presented to the emergency department with a 5-day history of progressively worsening general flu-like symptoms. He is currently in the emergency department's resuscitation bay. He is agitated and confused but with a patent airway. He has a respiratory rate of 24 breaths per minute, with an oxygen saturation of 96% on 15L of oxygen via a non-rebreathe reservoir mask.

1) On arrival you are presented with the following blood gas result (● Table 4.5). Please summarise this blood gas result.

1 mark
(0.5 mark for each correct stem)

Table 4.5. Arterial blood gas results.	
pH	7.11
PaO$_2$	11.2kPa
PaCO$_2$	3.2kPa
HCO$_3^-$	19mmol/L
Lactate	4.8mmol/L
BE	-5.4mmol/L

- Metabolic acidosis with partial respiratory compensation.
- Lactataemia.

2) List some other key clinical physiological markers that you should obtain.

1 mark
(0.25 mark for each correct stem)

- Heart rate.

- Mean arterial blood pressure (MAP).
- Capillary refill time.
- Temperature.

3) His heart rate is 102 beats per minute, the mean arterial blood pressure (MAP) 50mmHg, and the capillary refill is 5 seconds. The patient is febrile at 38.4°C. What is the definition of systemic inflammatory response syndrome (SIRS)?

2 marks
(0.5 mark for each correct stem)

The International Sepsis Definitions Conference proposed that SIRS can be diagnosed as having two out of the following four criteria:

- Temperature >38°C or <36°C.
- Heart rate >90 beats per minute.
- Respiratory rate >20 breaths per minute or $PaCO_2$ <4.3kPa.
- White blood cell count >12,000 cells/ml or <4000 cells/ml.

4) What guidance is widely used to manage sepsis?

0.5 mark

- The 2012 Surviving Sepsis Campaign.

5) List the components of the 3-hour and 6-hour care bundle.

The Surviving Sepsis Campaign (SSC) was created and subsequently updated in 2013 [1].

The first bundle is to be completed within the first 3 hours from clinical presentation:

2 marks
(0.5 mark for each correct stem)

- Measure plasma lactate level.
- Obtain blood cultures prior to administration of antibiotics.
- Administer broad-spectrum antibiotics.
- Administer 30ml/kg crystalloid for hypotension or lactate >4mmol/L.

The second care bundle is to be completed within 6 hours from clinical presentation:

2 marks
(0.5 mark for each correct stem)

- Infuse vasopressors to maintain a mean arterial pressure (MAP) of >65mmHg.
- In the event of persistent arterial hypotension, despite volume resuscitation (septic shock) or initial lactate >4mmol/L:
    - measure central venous pressure and target >8mmHg;
    - measure central venous oxygen saturation and target >70%.
- Remeasure lactate.

6) How can the circulatory status be assessed?

1.5 marks
(0.25 mark for each correct stem)

- Heart rate.
- Blood pressure.
- Urine output.
- Lactate.
- $ScvO_2$ (<70%).
- Cerebral perfusion (confusion, conscious level).

7) What specific investigations are necessary as part of a septic screen?

2 marks
(0.5 mark for each correct stem)

- Blood cultures, urinary and sputum samples for microscopy, culture, sensitivities (MC&S).
- Chest X-ray.
- Urinary pneumococcal antigen.
- Urinary *Legionella* antigen.

8) The patient has chest X-ray changes consistent with right-sided consolidation. There also appears to be a cavitating focal point. What antibiotics would you propose for this patient? Explain your rationale.

3 marks
(1 mark for each correct stem, with an example and reason for the cover)

- Intravenous antibiotics to include a:
  - beta-lactam — co-amoxiclav;
  - macrolide — clarithromycin for atypical micro-organism cover.
- The patient has septic shock; therefore, for bacteriocidal effect:
  - aminoglycocide — gentamicin.

9) You institute fluid resuscitation. What type of fluid would you choose and briefly outline how you have arrived at this choice?

- The choice of fluid advocated by the 2013 Surviving Sepsis Campaign is crystalloid which includes normal saline or Ringer's lactate solution [1].

0.5 mark

- Hydroxyethyl starch (HES) colloids are not advocated in sepsis.

0.5 mark

Trial evidence:

- The '6S' trial by Perner *et al* in 2012, a large multi-centred randomised controlled trial (RCT) comparing 6% HES with Ringer's lactate across 798 patients with severe sepsis [2]. The results found an increased risk of 90-day mortality with an increased requirement for renal replacement therapy in the HES group.
- A larger trial, the 'CHEST' trial, by Myburgh *et al* in 2012 was a multi-centred RCT comparing HES with 0.9% normal saline in the acute resuscitation of ICU patients [3]. 7000 patients were randomized, and there was no difference found in 90-day mortality but there was an increase in renal replacement requirements in the HES group.

1 mark
(for mentioning these two trials and the negative inference towards the use of HES)

- Albumin colloid has theoretical beneficial characteristics as a resuscitation fluid.
- The 'SAFE' trial in 2004 compared 4% albumin and normal saline in 6997 critically unwell patients [4]. 18% of the patients had severe sepsis. It was confirmed that albumin and normal saline had comparable 28-day mortality outcomes. However, patients with septic shock had a statistically non-significant trend towards a survival benefit with albumin.
- Hence, in the SSC 2013 guidelines there is a weak recommendation advocating the use of albumin in the resuscitation of septic shock when patients require substantial amounts of crystalloids.

1 mark
(for the suggestion of albumin, mention of the trial and when albumin should be used)

10) What are the elements of early goal-directed therapy (EGDT)?

1 mark

- CVP 8-12mmHg.
- MAP 65-90mmHg.

- Urine output >0.5ml/kg/hr.
- Mixed venous oxygen saturation >65% or mixed central oxygen saturation >70%.
- Haematocrit >30%.

11) What is the evidence for EGDT?

1 mark
(0.5 mark for each correct stem)

- The original Rivers study had limitations [5].
- Since then there have been three large multi-centred studies including the:
  - Australian/New Zealand ARISE [6];
  - UK ProMISE trial which looked at protocol-driven EGDT versus non-protocol-driven care [7];
  - US-based ProCESS study [8].

References

1. Dellinger RP, Mitchell ML, Rhodes A, *et al*. Surviving Sepsis Campaign: international guidelines for management of severe sepsis and septic shock, 2012. *Intensive Care Med* 2013; 39(2): 165-228.

2. Perner A, Haase N, Guttormsen AB, *et al*. Hydroxyethyl starch 130/0.42 versus Ringer's acetate in severe sepsis. *New Engl J Med* 2012; 367(2): 124-34.

3. Myburgh JA, Finfer S, Bellomo R, *et al*; CHEST Investigators. Australian and New Zealand Intensive Care Society Clinical Trials Group. Hydroxyethyl starch or saline for fluid resuscitation in intensive care. *N Engl J Med* 2012; 367(20): 1901-11.

4. Finfer S, Bellomo R, Boyce N, *et al*; SAFE Study Investigators. A comparison of albumin and saline for fluid resuscitation in the intensive care unit. *N Engl J Med* 2004; 350(22): 2247-56.

5. Rivers E, Nguyen B, Havstad S, *et al*. Early goal-directed therapy in the treatment of severe sepsis and septic shock. *N Engl J Med* 2001; 345(19): 1368-77.

Top Tip

The ProCESS trial is a randomised controlled multi-centred trial in 31 academic hospitals. The 1341 patients were randomised in a 1:1:1 ratio to protocolised early goal-directed therapy, protocolised standard therapy or usual care. The protocolised standard therapy used a lower haemoglobin threshold of 7.5g/dL. The use of ScvO₂ was discouraged. The primary endpoint of 60-day hospital mortality was not different across all three groups. The standard therapy group received less blood transfusion compared to the EGDT group (8.3% compared to 14.4%).

The ProMISE randomised controlled trial compared EGDT for the first 6 hours of management (n=630) with usual care (n=630), in 1260 patients with early septic shock across 56 UK hospitals. There was no difference in 90-day mortality, worse SOFA scores in the EGDT group and increased resource use in the EGDT group.

6.   Peake SL, Delaney A, Bailey M, *et al*; ARISE Investigators; ANZICS Clinical Trials Group. Goal-directed resuscitation for patients with early septic shock. *N Engl J Med* 2014; 371(16): 1496-506.

7.   Mouncey PR, Osborn TM, Power GS; ProMISe Trial Investigators. Trial of early, goal-directed resuscitation for septic shock. *N Engl J Med* 2015; 372: 1301-11.

8.   ProCESS investigators. A randomized trial of protocol-based care for early septic shock. *N Engl J Med* 2014; 370(18): 1683-93.

Refeeding syndrome

1) Please present this chest X-ray (Figure 4.4). 2 marks
(0.5 mark for
each correct
stem)

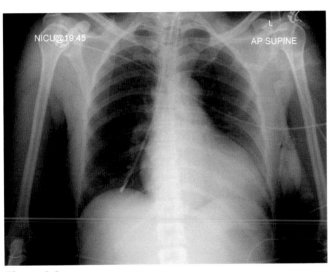

Figure 4.4.

- This is a plain AP film.
- An NG tube is sited in the right main bronchus.
- Loss of the left costophrenic angle.
- ECG leads are present.

2) Would you feed this patient? 1 mark

- No.

3) **Are you aware of any guidelines regarding feeding and misplaced NG tubes?**   2 marks

- The National Patient Safety Agency (NPSA) issued a patient safety alert in 2011, with the dangers of NG tube misplacement and feeding.
- This is classed as a 'never event'. Trusts have to put local policies in place to ensure that these events do not happen.

4) **How would you calculate the calorific requirements of a patient on the ICU? What are the problems with such calculations?**   2 marks (1 mark for each correct stem, with a maximum of 2 marks)

- BMI is a useful indicator.
- Schofield equation.
- They do not account for changes in the basal metabolic rate.

5) **What are the approximate daily requirements of calories, protein and fluid?**   3 marks

- Carbohydrate 25-35kcal/kg/day.
- Fluid 30-35ml/kg/day.
- Protein 0.8-1.5g/kg/day.

6) **You are presented with the following blood tests (● Table 4.6). Please summarise the abnormalities and suggest differential diagnoses.**   2 marks

Table 4.6. **Blood test results.**

Na$^+$	135mmol/L
K$^+$	2.3mmol/L
Cl$^-$	110mmol/L
HCO$_3^-$	25mmol/L
PO$_4$	1.2mmol/L
Mg	0.7mmol/L
Urea	7.8mmol/L
Creatinine	80µmol/L

- Hypokalaemia, hypomagnesaemia, hypophosphataemia.
- The results are consistent with refeeding syndrome.

7) What is the pathophysiology of refeeding syndrome? 3 marks

- Potassium, magnesium and phosphate are moved intracellularly after a sudden carbohydrate load.
- Associated with cardiac, respiratory and neurological complications.

8) How would you avoid/treat refeeding syndrome? 3 marks

Identify patients at risk:

- Patients with little or no feeding >5 days at risk.
- Alcoholics.
- Patients on drugs such as insulin, chemotherapy, antacids and diuretics.

NICE guidelines: 2 marks

- Commence feeding at 50% of usual requirements for 2 days, then increase by 200-400kcal per day.
- Appropriate micronutrient supplementation.
- Careful monitoring of electrolytes.

References

1. Mehanna HM, Moledina J, Travis J. Refeeding syndrome: what it is, and how to prevent and treat it. *BMJ* 2008; 336(7659): 1495-8.

SIADH, cerebral salt wasting and DI

A 32-year-old man involved in a high-speed motor-vehicle accident is at day 4 on the neuro-ICU. He was a motor-cyclist in a head-on collision with a concrete structure, which he hit trying to avoid a pedestrian who had suddenly walked into the road.

He received emergency neurosurgical intervention to evacuate an extradural haemorrhage. He had suffered some significant cerebral contusions in keeping with an overall moderate to severe traumatic brain injury. Other injuries included some minor fractures to his upper limbs and ribs.

Over the past 24 hours he has been assessed for extubation. However, his motor score of 6, where the patient had started to obey commands, has deteriorated to localising to pain, with significant agitation noticed during his last sedation hold. It is noticed that his mild hyponatraemia of 129mmol/L has significantly deteriorated and is now 118mmol/L.

1) How is sodium regulated in the body?

2 marks
(1 mark for each correct stem, with a maximum of 2 marks)

- Sodium is the major extracellular cation.
- The intracellular to extracellular concentration gradient is maintained by the sodium-potassium ATPase pump.
- Total body sodium is regulated by renal excretion — under hormonal influence, for example, brain natriuretic peptide (BNP).

2) What is the normal value for plasma osmolality?   0.5 mark

- 285-295mOsm/kg.

3) In this case what are your potential differential diagnoses for hyponatraemia?   2 marks

- Cerebral salt wasting syndrome (CSWS).
- Syndrome of inappropriate antidiuretic hormone (ADH) secretion (SIADH).

4) What specific investigations would you order to help differentiate hyponatraemia between CSWS and SIADH?   2 marks (0.5 mark for each correct stem)

- Serum sodium.
- Serum osmolality.
- Urine sodium.
- Urine osmolality.

A comment about being paired samples should be made.

5) Serum and urine osmolalities are requested and the following results are obtained (● Table 4.7). What additional clinical information would you require to supplement this biochemical data?   2 marks

Table 4.7. Urinary and serum sodium and osmolalities.

Serum Na$^+$	117mmol/L
Serum osmolality	242mOsm/kg
	(285-295mOsm/kg)
Urine Na$^+$	26mmol/L
Urine osmolality	1223mOsm/kg
	(500-800mOsm/kg)

- Volume status of the patient — if the patient is euvolaemic, hypovolaemic, or dehydrated.
- Urine output — oligoanuric with concentrated urine, or normal amounts of urine.

6) On reviewing the ICU chart you find the following clinical parameters (●Table 4.8). What is the most likely diagnosis?

1 mark

Table 4.8. Clinical parameters.

HR	88 bpm
BP	146/87mmHg
Capillary refill time	<2 seconds
CVP	14cmH$_2$0
Fluid balance for the last 24 hours is positive 2.2L	
The patient does not appear dehydrated	

- The likely diagnosis is SIADH as opposed to CSWS.

7) What factors will influence your management plan for the hyponatraemia?   3 marks

The determinants of how quickly the hyponatraemia should be managed is based on:

- The rate of fall of Na^+.
- The degree of hyponatraemia.
- If the patient has attributable symptomology to the hyponatraemia:
  - agitation, confusion, fluctuations in consciousness, seizures, coma.

8) What management should be instituted for this particular patient and why?   3 marks

- This patient has had a rapid fall in Na^+ and is now symptomatic as well.
- Although fluid restriction is the mainstay of management, allowing a steady rise in serum Na^+, in this case 1.8% or 3% hypertonic saline should be given as the patient is compromised.
- Once Na^+ levels reach 125mmol/L the hypertonic saline should be stopped and fluid restriction continued.

9) What is the risk of rapidly correcting a hyponatraemia?   0.5 mark

- Central pontine myolinolysis.

10) Name two other pharmacological measures and describe their mechanism of action in the management of SIADH.

2 marks

- Demeclocycline — functions as an antagonist to the actions of ADH by inhibiting the renal fluid retention capabilities of ADH.
- ADH-receptor antagonists — for example, lixivaptan, which acts as a direct antagonist to ADH.

11) Three days on from this incident the patient suddenly starts to produce large amounts of urine. In the subsequent 12-hour period the patient becomes 3.8L negative. Once again paired urinary and serum sodium and osmolalities are obtained (●Table 4.9). What is the likely cause of this change in urinary output?

1 mark

Table 4.9. Urinary and serum sodium and osmolalities.

Serum Na$^+$	151mmol/L
Serum osmolality	309mOsm/kg
	(285-295mOsm/kg)
Urine Na$^+$	26mmol/L
Urine osmolality	310mOsm/kg
	(500-800mOsm/kg)

- Diabetes insipidus.

12) How would you manage this condition?

1 mark

(0.5 mark for each correct stem)

- Prompt fluid resuscitation.
- Administration of synthetic ADH — desmopressin (DDAVP).

References

1. Bradshaw K, Smith M. Disorders of sodium balance after brain injury. *Contin Educ Anaesth Crit Care Pain* 2008; 8(4): 129-33.

Subarachnoid haemorrhage

You are the ICU doctor and are called to the emergency department's resuscitation area to see a 56-year-old man who has been admitted following a seizure at home.

He is not known to be epileptic, and other than hypertension he has no other medical conditions.

On your arrival he is no longer seizing and the nursing staff state that his GCS is 12/15.

1) Outline your initial management.

3 marks

(1 mark for each correct stem, with a maximum of 3 marks)

- Acute assessment, resuscitation and management should be undertaken to follow an 'airway, breathing, circulation, disability and exposure' approach.
- Apply high-flow oxygen.
- Obtain a set of observations.
- Ensure venous access and blood is sent for testing (FBC/U&Es/coagulation profile/LFT/CRP).
- Gather collateral history.

2) Whilst you are undertaking these tasks you notice that he is no longer speaking, you assess his GCS and find that it is now 8/15. What is the next step in your management?

2 marks

(1 mark for each correct stem, with a maximum of 2 marks)

- Intubation.
- Using a rapid sequence induction.
- This patient needs an urgent CT of the head.

3) You accompany the patient to the CT scanner   4 marks
   and the following image is obtained (● Figure
   4.5). What does this CT scan show?

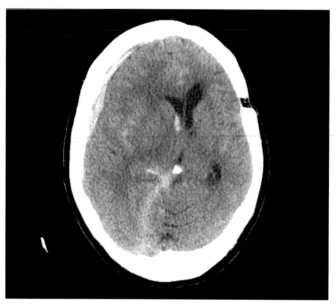

Figure 4.5.

- Acute subarachnoid haemorrhage (SAH).
- Small subdural haemorrhage.
- Intraventricular blood.
- Significant mid-line shift.

4) How would you classify subarachnoid   1 mark
   haemorrhage?

- Clinical or radiological.

5) Please outline a classification system.

4 marks
(marks for one of the 2 classifications)

● World Federation of Neurosurgeons (1998) (● Table 4.10.

Table 4.10. World Federation of Neurosurgeons classification of SAH.

I	GCS 15, no motor deficit.
II	GCS 13-14, no motor deficit.
III	GCS 13-14, motor deficit.
IV	GCS 7-12 +/- motor deficit.
V	GCS 3-6, motor deficit present or absent.

● Fisher (1980) (● Table 4.11).

Table 4.11. Fisher classification of SAH.

I	No blood.
II	Diffuse deposition of SAH without clots or layers of blood >1mm.
III	Localized clots and/or vertical layers of blood 1mm or > thickness.
IV	Diffuse or no subarachnoid blood but intracerebral or intraventricular clots.

Top
Tip

In the exam when asked for a classification system it is likely they will only have one on the mark sheet. Before you embark on wasting precious time outlining a system for which you will gain no marks, it is worth naming the system and enquiring as to whether this is the system they want. You should be told to "name another one" if your system is not on the mark sheet!

6) How would you manage this patient?

The patient should be managed in a critical care environment and ideally in a tertiary neurosurgical centre.   1 mark

The principle of initial management involves the prevention of further brain injury: 2 marks (0.5 mark for each correct stem, with a maximum of 2 marks)

- Mechanical ventilation — maintain a normal $PaCO_2$.
- Invasive arterial blood pressure monitoring and systolic pressure <180mmHg (MAP <110mmHg).
- Maintain normoglycaemia.
- Nurse at 45° in a head-up position.
- Avoid tight endotracheal tube ties.

7)   What are the complications of subarachnoid haemorrhage?

3 marks
(0.5 mark for each correct stem)

- Rebleeding.
- Seizures.
- Vasospasm.
- Hydrocephalus.
- Adrenergic 'storm'.
- Electrolyte imbalances (particularly sodium).

References

1.   Luoma A., Reddy U. Acute management of aneurysmal subarachnoid haemorrhage. *Cont Educ Anaesth Crit Care Pain* 2013; 13(2): 52-8.

Tetanus

You are asked to review a 32-year-old unkempt gentleman with a longstanding history of intravenous drug use (IVDU). The patient is very agitated and appears to have great difficulty breathing. The emergency department doctor has concerns with his airway as he appears to be having jaw and neck muscular spasms. The patient has severe pain brought on by the spasms, which seem to be precipitated by minimal stressors such as loud noises or anxiety.

1) The following blood results have been obtained (● Table 4.12). What is the most likely diagnosis?   1 mark

Table 4.12. Blood test results.	
Hb	94g/L
WCC	13 x 10⁹/L
Platelets	310 x 10⁹/L
Urea	8.2mmol/L
Creatinine	122μmol/L
CRP	210mg/L
Calcium	2.10mmol/L

● Tetanus.

(It cannot be tetany secondary to hypocalcaemia, as the calcium level is normal.)

2) What is tetanus? Please explain the pathophysiology of the condition.

4 marks
(1 mark for each correct stem, with a maximum of 4 marks)

- Tetanus is a neurological condition caused by infection by *Clostridium tetani*.
- The spores are found in the soil, and enter the body via broken skin.
- On entry into the body, a potent neurotoxin called tetanospasmin is released.
- Tetanospasmin targets the central nervous system particularly the neuromuscular junction.
- It spreads to affect motor and autonomic nervous activity.
- Tetanospasmin binds irreversibly and blocks inhibitory neurotransmitters such as glycine or GABA, hence the unopposed motor activity with life-critical autonomic activity.

3) What autonomic features are characteristically seen in tetanus?

3 marks

- Sympathetic 'storming' — hypertension, tachycardia, associated dysrhythmias.
- Sudden cardiovascular collapse — hypotension, bradycardia, bradyarrhythmias disseminating into asystole.
- Other features of unopposed sympathetic autonomic stimulation — such as sweating, hypersecretions and hyperpyrexia.

4) Why does a patient with tetanus require critical care admission?

4 marks

(1 mark for each correct stem, with a maximum of 4 marks)

- Critical care — high dependency care may escalate to ICU care for organ support.
- Quiet, calm and dark environment.
- Provision of multimodal analgesia and sedation.
- Vigilant advanced monitoring for autonomic disturbances.
- Organ support including ventilator support, vasopressor and/or inotropic support.

5) In addition to critical care admission what are the specific key management principles in tetanus?

- Acute control of muscular spasm: 0.5 mark
  - benzodiazipines and opiate (morphine)-based analgesia; 0.5 mark
  - sedation — propofol; 0.5 mark
  - other agents that can be considered — anticonvulsants or dantrolene; 0.5 mark
  - muscle relaxation for resistant muscular spasm. 0.5 mark
- Surgical wound debridement. 0.5 mark
- Antimicrobial therapy — metronidazole IV. 1 mark (for both)
- Human tetanus immunoglobulins — these will not affect the tetanospasmin already neuronally attached. However, they can prevent further progression. 1 mark
- Active and passive immunisation, i.e tetanus vaccine as well. 1 mark
- Autonomic instability: 0.5 mark
  - gain control through sedation and analgesia; 0.5 mark
  - magnesium sulphate — dampens down the sympathetic cascade; 0.5 mark

- sudden cardiovascular collapse can occur   0.5 mark
  swiftly after an intense sympathetic 'storm'.
  Unopposed vagal or parasympathetic activity
  may require urgent atropine.

References

1.   Taylor AM. Tetanus. *Contin Educ Anaesth Crit Care Pain* 2006;
   6(3): 101-4.

Equipment

1) What is this piece of equipment (● Figure 4.6)   2 marks
   and what is it used for?

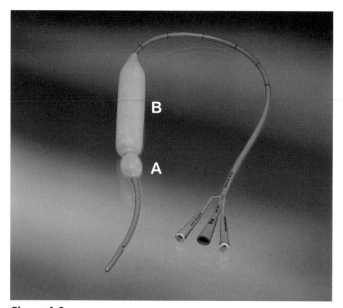

Figure 4.6.

- Sengstaken-Blakemore tube.
- It is used to tamponade oesophageal/gastric varices that are refractory to medical/endoscopic therapy.

2) Please identify the following parts labelled A   2 marks
   and B.

- A — gastric balloon.

- B — oesophageal balloon.

3) **What are the contraindications for using this piece of equipment?**   2 marks

- Known oesophageal stricture.
- Recent oesophageal surgery.

4) **How would you insert this piece of equipment?**   8 marks
(0.5 mark for each correct stem)

Preparation:

- The patient's best interests should be taken into account and a valid consent obtained.
- Consideration of airway protection (most patients are intubated for this procedure).
- Local anaesthetic jelly to nostril +/- vasoconstrictor (e.g. ephedrine drops).
- The patient is placed in a semi-recumbent position at 45°.
- Test and lubricate balloons.

Insertion:

- Introduce through the nostril or mouth.
- Insert to at least the 50cm markings.
- May need to use direct laryngoscopy to pass the tube into the oesophagus.
- Confirm the position of the gastric balloon with CXR.

Inflation:

- Always inflate the gastric balloon first.
- Inflate in a stepwise fashion with 50ml aliquots of air.
- Inflate up to 250-300ml.
- Pull the balloon up to the gastric fundus.
- Note the length at the lips.
- Attach to the traction system (e.g. 500ml bag of fluid).
- May need to inflate the oesophageal balloon, but this is often not required.

5) What are the complications of using this piece of equipment?

4 marks
(1 mark for each correct stem, with a maximum of 4 marks)

- Pain.
- Haemorrhage.
- Oesophageal or gastric rupture.
- Pressure necrosis.
- Upper airway obstruction.

6) How can you minimise the risk of pressure necrosis?

2 marks

- Limit the time that the balloon(s) is inflated.
- Only use the tube for 24 hours.

Electrocardiography — set 4

1) This is an electrocardiogram (ECG) of a 54-year-old lady (● Figure 4.7). Please describe this ECG.

3 marks
(0.5 mark for each correct stem, with a maximum of 3 marks)

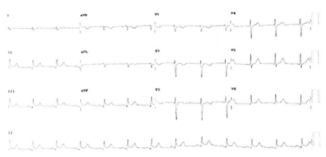

Figure 4.7.

- Rate — 75 beats per minute.
- Rhythm — regular rhythm.
- Axis — normal axis.
- P-wave morphology and P-R interval — P-waves have a normal morphology with a normal P-R interval.
- QRS complex — normal QRS complex.
- ST segments — ST elevation in II, III and aVF.
- T-wave morphology — T-wave inversion V1, V2 and V3.

2) What is the diagnosis?

- Inferior ST elevation myocardial infarction.

1 mark

3) **How would you manage this patient if they had chest pain?** 2 marks

- Acute assessment, resuscitation and management should be undertaken to follow an 'airway, breathing, circulation, disability and exposure' approach.
- The patient will require urgent referral for a cardiology review for revascularisation options to be instituted — percutaneous coronary intervention (PCI) or thrombolysis.

4) **What is the most common complication with an inferior territory myocardial infarction and why?** 2 marks

- Cardiac dysrhythmias, for example, complete heart block.
- The infarct in this territory can render ischaemic compromise to the sinoatrial node (SAN) and atrioventricular node (AVN) axis; hence there is a vulnerability to cardiac dysrhythmias.

5) **This ECG belongs to a 49-year-old lady who was awaiting a session of dialysis which she normally receives three times a week (● Figure 4.8). Please describe this ECG.** 3 marks
(0.5 mark for each correct stem, with a maximum of 3 marks)

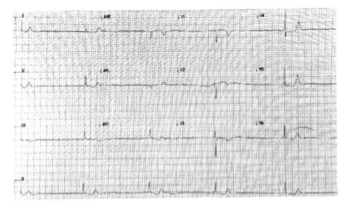

Figure 4.8.

- Rate — 30 beats a minute.
- Rhythm — the ventricular rhythm seen is regular.
- Axis — normal axis.
- P-wave morphology and P-R interval — P-waves are not clearly and consistently seen, hence the P-R interval is indiscernible.
- QRS complex — normal QRS complex.
- ST segments — isoelectric.
- T-wave morphology — T-wave inversion in V1, V2 and V3.

6)   What is the diagnosis?   2 marks

- Ventricular escape rhythm with no atrial activity, hence severe bradycardia.

7) What would be your management strategies and options if the patient was hypotensive with this ECG?

- Acute assessment, resuscitation and management should be undertaken to follow an 'airway, breathing, circulation, disability and exposure' approach.   1 mark

- Attach the patient to the defibrillator and monitor the heart rate and rhythm via the paddles.   1 mark

- The defibrillator can be set to deliver transcutaneous pacing.   1 mark

- Pharmacological options to increase the heart rate include: 2 marks
  - atropine 600µg intravenously (IV) as an initial dose;
  - isoprenaline as an IV infusion;
  - consideration of adrenaline.

- Transcutaneous pacing options should be sought concurrently with an urgent cardiological review for: 1 mark
  - a temporary pacing wire;
  - possible permanent pacing systems.

- The underlying cause should be sought and reversed if possible, for example, severe hyperkalaemia which has caused a deterioration in the ECG rhythm.   1 mark

Radiology — set 4

1) Please present this chest X-ray (● Figure 4.9). 5 marks

(1 mark for each correct stem, with a maximum of 5 marks)

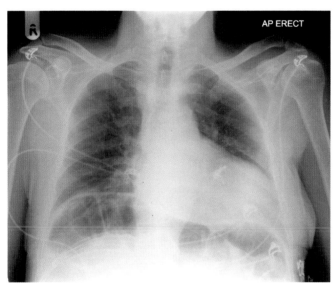

Figure 4.9.

- AP chest X-ray film.
- Slightly under-penetrated.
- Increased vascular markings in both lung fields.
- Dilated transverse colon, but no free air.
- ECG leads.
- Large cardiac shadow.

2) Please present the following X-ray (● Figure 4.10).

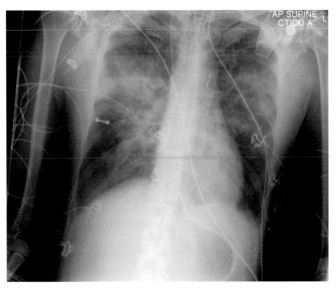

Figure 4.10.

● AP chest film.	3 marks
● Adequate penetration.	(1 mark for each
● Peri-hilar shadowing, consistent with pulmonary oedema.	correct stem, with a maximum
● Some blunting of the left costophrenic angle.	of 3 marks)
ICU paraphernalia:	6 marks
	(1 mark for each
● Intra-aortic balloon pump.	correct stem,
● Nasogastric tube, adequate position.	with a maximum
● Right internal jugular central venous catheter.	of 6 marks)
● Endotracheal tube.	
● ECG electrodes.	

- Syringe attached to in-line closed suction.
- Left nipple piercing (no marks for this!).

3) Please present the following X-ray (● Figure 4.11).

6 marks
(1 mark for each correct stem, with a maximum of 6 marks)

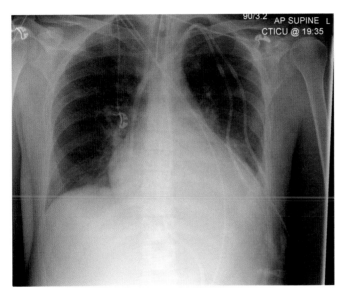

Figure 4.11.

- AP chest film.
- Adequate penetration.
- Increased peri-hilar vascular markings.
- Loss of left costophrenic angle, likely to represent a pleural effusion.
- Large cardiac shadow.
- Tunnelled dialysis line.
- Endotracheal tube.
- ECG electrodes.

Top Tip

You should have a systematic system for presenting images. You will need to mention the specific points on the examiner's mark sheet to gain the mark. You may see (or think you see!) other abnormalities on the X-rays but you will only gain marks for what is on the sheet.

Chapter 5

Trauma — massive blood transfusion

A 22-year-old man is brought to the emergency department having sustained significant trauma. He had been attacked and beaten by a group of men, and then ran over by a vehicle. He has marked tenderness in the abdomen and appears to be agitated and combatant. There is no history or evidence of alcohol or substance intake. He has not received formal pre-hospital care and was found left outside the hospital.

Amongst his injuries the patient has bruising across his chest and left flank with marked abdominal tenderness on examination. He has open fractures of his left leg and a traumatic amputation of his right leg distal to the knee. A belt had been tied as a make-shift tourniquet high above the right knee. His bedside observations are detailed below in ● Table 5.1.

Table 5.1. Observations.

Respiratory rate	24 breaths per minute
SaO_2	98% on room air
BP	75/34mmHg
HR	122 bpm
Capillary refill time	4.5 seconds
GCS	E 4 V 3 M 5

1) How would you approach this patient's management?

1 mark
(must state or address catastrophic haemorrhage)

An approach following a:

- Catastrophic haemorrhage.
- C-Spine and airway.
- Breathing.
- Circulation.
- Disability.

2) A blood gas analysis is undertaken and the results are detailed below in ● Table 5.2. Please summarise the results.

2 marks
(1 mark for each correct stem)

Table 5.2. Arterial blood gas results.

pH	7.28
PaO$_2$	13.7kPa
PaCO$_2$	3.4kPa
HCO$_3^-$	20.2mmol/L
Cl$^-$	87mmol/L
Lactate	4.7mmol/L
BE	-6.8mmol/L
Hb	68g/L

- A metabolic acidosis with attempted respiratory compensation, and a raised lactate.
- Profound anaemia.

3) **What principle of resuscitation would you employ for this patient?** 1 mark

- The patient requires blood product resuscitation.

4) **What options for access for fluid therapy do you have in this patient?** 3 marks (1 mark for each correct stem)

- IV access — two large-bore cannulae.
- If this is at all difficult to establish then swiftly secure intraosseous access.
- If the skill set is present then large-gauge central venous access should be instigated, for example, using a 8.5-gauge trauma line or a 'Swan' sheath/PA catheter introducer.

5) **The patient has a tibial intraosseous and one 16g IV access established. What fluid resuscitation would you implement?** 3 marks (1 mark for each correct stem; must state ratio for PRBCs:FFP; No negative marking if crystalloid transfusion stated)

- Requires packed red blood cells (PRBCs) and fresh frozen plasma (FFP) transfused at a 1:1 or 2:1 ratio.
- Platelets may be required early.
- Crystalloids should be avoided and blood products used.
- Cryoprecipitate may be required.

6) **You are presented with the following picture (● Figure 5.1). What is this piece of data? Please interpret it.** 6 marks (1 mark for each correct stem)

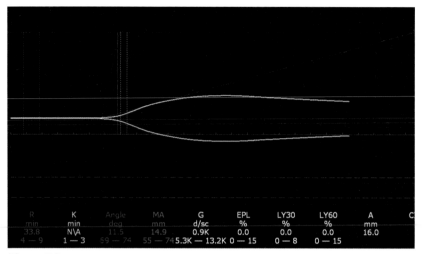

R	K	Angle	MA	G	EPL	LY30	LY60	A	C
min	min	deg	mm	d/sc	%	%	%	mm	
33.8	N\A	11.5	14.9	0.9K	0.0	0.0	0.0	16.0	
4 — 9	1 — 3	59 — 74	55 — 74	5.3K — 13.2K	0 — 15	0 — 8	0 — 15		

Figure 5.1.

- This is a thromboelastography (TEG®) image.
- The R-time is prolonged — indicating a decreased level of coagulation factors.
- The K-time is unrecordable — indicating either a sampling error OR deficiency in clotting factors, platelets and fibrinogen, as this is a marker of clot formation dynamics.
- The α-angle is decreased — this indicates that the rate at which the clot is forming is significantly slowed down.
- The maximum amplitude is decreased — this indicates a low platelet count OR poor platelet function.
- The shape of the curve is starting to taper off indicating abnormal fibrinolysis, with likely low fibrinogen and platelets.

7) What other measures can be taken to address a coagulopathy of trauma?

4 marks

(1 mark for each correct stem, with a maximum of 4 marks. Must mention at least 2 examples for stopping the bleeding)

- Stop the bleeding — direct pressure, tourniquets, surgery, embolisation.
- Avoid crystalloid fluid resuscitation, and if used avoid large volumes.
- Regular near-bed-side analysis of coagulation such as TEG® or rotational thromboelastometry (ROTEM®).
- Tranexamic acid — initial bolus 1g over 10 minutes followed by an infusion of 1g over 8 hours.

(must recognise that 2 doses are given)

- Prevent or correct acidosis.
- Prevent or correct hypothermia.
- Calcium chloride — particularly if <0.8mmol/L.

References

1. Srivastava A, Kelleher A. Point-of-care coagulation testing. *Cont Educ Anaesth Crit Care Pain* 2013; 13(1): 12-6.

Stroke

You are the doctor on-call for the ICU and are called to see a 62-year-old woman brought into the emergency department. She was found collapsed on the floor by her husband, who called the ambulance. Initially she was confused but on arrival her Glasgow Coma Scale (GCS) score dropped and is now 7/15. She has a past medical history of type 2 diabetes and hypertension.

1) Please outline your initial management.

4 marks

(0.5 mark for each correct stem)

- Acute assessment, resuscitation and management should be undertaken to follow an 'airway, breathing, circulation, disability and exposure' approach.
- Assess GCS and airway.
- Apply monitoring.
- Gain intravenous access.
- Send bloods for standard tests but to include a toxicology screen.
- Measures to secure the airway should be made.
- Intubation should be by a rapid sequence induction (RSI).
- This patient will need an urgent CT scan of her brain.

2) The patient is intubated and taken for a CT of the head. What does the CT show (● Figure 5.2)?

2 marks

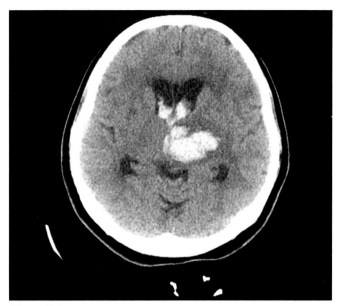

Figure 5.2.

- There is a haemorrhagic stroke within the basal ganglia, with evidence of intraventricular haemorrhage.

3) What is the likely cause of this?   1 mark

- Hypertension.

4) How are strokes classified?   3 marks
(1 mark for naming the classification and 2 marks in total for correctly naming the four types)

- Oxford Stroke Classification (also known as the Bamford Classification). These are classified into four types based on symptoms (● Table 5.3).

Table 5.3. Oxford Stroke Classification.

TACS	Total anterior circulation stroke
PACS	Partial anterior circulation syndrome
POCS	Posterior circulation syndrome
LACS	Lacunar syndrome

5) Can you describe the National Institutes of Health Stroke Scale (NIHSS)?

4 marks
(1 mark for each correct stem, with a maximum of 4 marks)

- This is a system to assess the severity of an acute stroke and there are 11 domains tested.
- The combination of the scores from each domain gives a final score.
- This is a good predictor of patient outcome.
- A score >16 indicates a strong possibility of death.
- A score <6 indicates the likelihood of a good recovery.

(Other scoring systems do exist, e.g. ABCD2 and CHADS2.)

6) When considering the NIHSS what are the maximum and minimum values?

1 mark

- 0 = no stroke.
- 42 = severe stroke.

7) What complications is this patient at risk from?

4 marks

- Further bleeding.

- Hydrocephalus and vasospasm due to the presence of intraventricular blood.
- Oedema leading to raised ICP.
- Seizures.

8) How would you manage this patient's blood pressure?

1 mark

- The ATACH (Antihypertensive Treatment of Acute Cerebral Haemorrhage) and INTERACT (Intensive Blood Pressure Reduction in Acute Cerebral Haemorrhage Trial) trials have shown that maintaining a systolic blood pressure <140mmHg is associated with less haematoma expansion. The effect on outcome is less clear.

References

1.   Raithatha A, Pratt G, Rash A. Developments in the management of acute ischaemic stroke: implications for anaesthetic and critical care management. *Cont Educ Anaesth Crit Care Pain* 2013; 13(3): 80-6.

Trauma — diaphragmatic rupture

You are asked to review a 32-year-old male who has presented to the emergency department with significant dyspnoea. He has been involved in a high-speed road traffic accident. He was the driver in a vehicle, restrained in his seat by the seatbelt. The airbag had not deployed.

1) You are presented with the following X-ray image taken 5 days after admission (● Figure 5.3). Please present this film.

3 marks

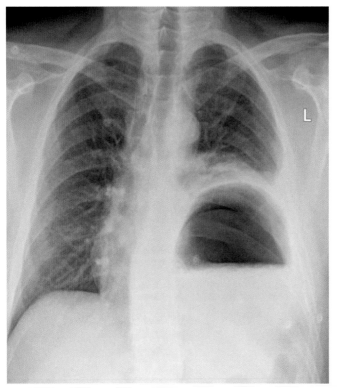

Figure 5.3.

- This is a chest radiograph.
- There is a large gastric air-fluid level in the lower half of the left hemithorax.
- The mediastinal structures including the heart are displaced to the right.

2) What other imaging modality would you request?   1 mark

- CT of the thorax and abdomen.

3) What is the likely diagnosis?   1 mark

- This is likely to be a traumatic herniation of abdominal structures through a ruptured diaphragm.

(If the candidate fails to identify the correct diagnosis please inform them that this is a diaphragmatic rupture.)

4) What percentage of cases are missed on an initial chest radiograph?   1 mark (accept anything between 40-60% as an answer)

- 50% are missed on CXRs.

5) Which side of the chest is most commonly affected and by what proportion?   1 mark (0.5 mark for the correct side and 0.5 mark for the proportion)

- There is a three-times greater proportion of traumatic diaphragmatic herniation on the left side compared to the right hemi-diaphragm.

6) How would you manage a patient with a   2 marks
   diaphragmatic rupture?

This patient should be managed as follows:

- C-spine, and the 'airway, breathing, circulation, disability and exposure' approach as per the ATLS guidelines.
- Specifically, the patient requires a surgical review.

7) What proportion require surgical intervention?   1 mark

- 100% of cases require surgical repair.

8) What other key organ structures could have   2 marks
   been damaged with blunt trauma based on   (0.5 mark for
   the above case of left-sided diaphragmatic   each correct
   rupture?   stem, with a
       maximum of 2
- Cardiac and great vessel structures.   marks)
- Pulmonary structures.
- Splenic rupture.
- Right kidney.
- Bowel — large and small bowel

9) A splenic rupture is diagnosed. Are you aware   4 marks
   of a classification system for this diagnosis?   (1 mark for
       each correct
The American Association for the Surgery of Trauma   stem, with a
Organ Injury Scale: maximum of 4
       marks)
- Grades I-V.

- Is based on a number of factors including:
  - the state of the vascular structures;
  - the surface area of the haematoma size;
  - the laceration size.

10) How would you manage a splenic injury?

4 marks

(1 mark for each correct stem, with a maximum of 4 marks)

- Catastrophic haemorrhage control following the 'airway, breathing, circulation, disability and exposure' approach — with particular note to the cardiovascular status.
- Grade I-III injuries can often be managed conservatively with no surgical or radiological intervention.
- Grade IV-V injuries require urgent intervention.
- Interventional radiology with embolisation.
- Emergency surgery for splenectomy may be required.

References

1. Sohini S, Shirley P. Trauma anaesthesia and critical care: the post trauma network era. *Cont Educ Anaesth Crit Care Pain* 2014; 14(1): 32-7.

2. Tinkoff G, Esposito TJ, Reed J, *et al*. American Association for the Surgery of Trauma Organ Injury Scale I: spleen, liver, and kidney, validation based on the National Trauma Data Bank. *J Am Coll Surg* 2008; 207(5): 646-55.

3. Liu PP, Liu HT, Hsieh TM, *et al*. Nonsurgical management of delayed splenic rupture after blunt trauma. *J Trauma Acute Care Surg* 2012; 72(4): 1019-23.

Thrombotic thrombocytopaenic purpura in pregnancy

You are asked to review a patient in the labour ward HDU. She is 32 weeks pregnant and has been complaining of increasing shortness of breath over the past 2 days. She contacted her community midwife and was asked to attend the emergency department where she was quickly transferred to the labour ward.

When you arrive she is mildly confused with an Abbreviated Mental Test Score (AMTS) of 8, and has a temperature of 39.4°C. Her heart rate is 120 bpm and her blood pressure 115/76mmHg.

1) The obstetric team has sent off some blood for testing and the results are shown in ● Table 5.4. Please comment on the results.

2 marks
(0.5 mark for each correct stem, with a maximum of 2 marks)

Table 5.4. Blood test results.

Hb	80g/L
WCC	14.1×10^9/L
Platelets	22×10^9/L
Neutrophils	11×10^9/L
Reticulocytes	Seen on the blood film
INR	1.2
APTT	1.09
Na^+	135mmol/L
K^+	5.3mmol/L
Cl^-	110mmol/L
HCO_3	19mmol/L

Continued

Table 5.4. Blood test results *continued*.

Bilirubin	28μmol/L
Urea	23.5mmol/L
Creatinine	345μmol/L
LDH	834i.u./L
ALP	125i.u./L
AST	50i.u./L
GGT	68i.u./L
Albumin	35g/L
Amylase	50i.u./L
Troponin I	350ng/L

- Thrombocytopaenia.
- Acute kidney injury (AKI).
- Mildly deranged liver function.
- Raised troponin.
- High reticulocyte count.
- Raised inflammatory markers.

2) Please list your differential diagnoses.

3 marks
(0.5 mark for each correct stem, with a maximum of 3 marks)

- Thrombotic thrombocytopaenic purpura (TTP).
- Haemolytic uraemic syndrome.
- HELLP.
- Pre-eclampsia/eclampsia.
- Sepsis.
- Malignancy.
- Disseminated intravascular coagulation (DIC).
- Malignant hypertension.

3) What additional tests would you perform?

3 marks

(0.5 mark for each correct stem, with a maximum of 3 marks)

- Chest X-ray.
- ECG.
- Blood film.
- Hepatitis screen/HIV.
- Haptoglobins.
- ADAMTS13.
- Autoantibody screen.
- Thyroid function tests.
- Consider CT of the head.

4) A blood film is sent and the haematology doctor calls you to tell you that it shows red cell fragments consistent with microangiopathic haemolytic anaemia (MAHA). How would you manage this patient?

6 marks

- This patient has TTP, which is a haematological emergency.
- The patient requires immediate referral to a tertiary centre for specialist management.
- In the meantime treatment is supportive, which may include a transfusion of packed red cells and or FFP if clinically indicated.
- A platelet transfusion should NOT be given.
- Consider an emergency lower segment Caesarean section (LSCS).
- Consider giving steroids, both for the TTP and the foetus, but discuss this with the haematologist/obstetrician.

5) What is the pathophysiology behind TTP?   2 marks

- There are IgG antibodies formed against ADAMST13 (which is a von Willebrand cleaving protease). This leads to increased amounts of uncleaved von Willebrand factor which subsequently causes abnormal platelet aggregation and destruction, as well as a thrombotic phenomenon.

6) The patient is transferred to the nearest tertiary centre. How would a patient with TTP be managed?   4 marks

- Plasma exchange with 1.5x plasma volume, until the platelet count is >150 x 10^9/L for 2 consecutive days
- Methylprednisolone after first plasma exchange.
- When the platelet count is >50 x 10^9/L, consider starting low-molecular-weight heparin/aspirin.
- Rituximab is considered in patients who fail to respond to plasma exchange or steroids.

References

1.   Sadler JE. Von Willebrand factor, ADAMTS13, and thrombotic thrombocytopenic purpura. *Blood* 2008; 112(1): 11-8.

Traumatic brain injury and management of raised ICP

A 39-year-old gentleman is involved in a fight in a bar. He receives a single blow with a bottle to his head and instantly falls to the ground. When the paramedics arrive he is conscious but very agitated and combative. The patient is anaesthetised at the scene, intubated and ventilated, and subsequently flown by helicopter to the nearest trauma centre. During the flight it is noted that his left pupil is fixed and dilated. The crew administer hypertonic saline. On arrival you are called as part of the trauma team where he is taken straight to CT from the helipad.

1) Please describe the image below (● Figure 5.4).

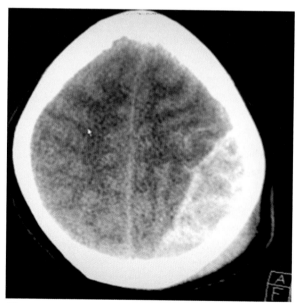

Figure 5.4.

- This is a CT of the head.   0.5 mark
- Large left-sided extradural haemorrhage.   1 mark
- Mass effect and some shift of the midline.   1 mark
- No space around the cortex visible, in keeping with a   0.5 mark
raised ICP.

2) What immediate measures would you take for   2 marks
this patient?

- Acute assessment, resuscitation and management should be undertaken to follow an 'airway, breathing, circulation, disability and exposure' approach.
- Appreciate that this is a neurosurgical emergency and urgent surgical decompression/evacuation of haemorrhage is required.

3) What specific breathing measures and targets would you aim for?

Whilst concurrently transferring the patient to theatre:

- Airway secured.   0.5 mark
- Breathing:
  - PaO_2 >10kPa;   0.5 mark
  - $PaCO_2$ 4.5-5.0kPa;   0.5 mark
  - hyperventilating the patient may risk ischaemia.   0.5 mark

If the candidate states a lower $PaCO_2$ this must be justified in that this would be a one-off manoeuvre to urgently decrease ICP as a life-saving measure.

4) What aims would you have for the circulation and what is the rationale?

- CPP = MAP - ICP: 1 mark
  - aim for CPP >60mmHg;   1 mark
  - avoid hypotension — aim for a MAP >90mmHg   1 mark
    (Brain Trauma Foundation).

5) What other measures should be considered?

Disability:

- Mannitol 0.5-1g/kg or hypertonic saline (5%) 1-   1 mark
  2ml/kg.
- Check pupils, the GCS and check for features of   1 mark
  coning.

Other general measures: 4 marks

(1 mark for

- Loosen any pressure around the neck; use tape for   each correct
  the endotracheal tube, not ties.   stem, with a
- Head-up positioning.   maximum of 4
- Low normothermia temperature <37°C.   marks)
- Blood sugar — aim for normoglycaemia — 6-
  10mmol/L.
- Urgent pharmacological intervention for any seizure
  activity.
- Deepen anaesthesia.

6) What other second-line therapies are available?

4 marks

(1 mark for

each correct

stem)

- Decompressive craniectomy.

- Hypothermia to 35°C.
- CSF drainage (external ventricular drain [EVD]).
- Barbiturate (thiopentone) coma.

References

1. Dinsmore J. Traumatic brain injury: an evidence-based review of management. *Cont Educ Anaesth Crit Care Pain* 2013; 13(6): 189-95.

Warfarin

You are asked to review an 82-year-old female in the emergency department who has presented following a mechanical fall at home. She has epistaxis, which is ongoing and has right-sided rib fractures on her chest X-ray.

1) Please describe the key features of the   2 marks
   following blood results (● Table 5.5).

Table 5.5. Blood test results.	
Hb	78g/L
WCC	12.1 x 10^9/L
Platelets	109 x 10^9/L
MCV	90fL
PT	32 seconds (10-12 secs)
aPTT	0.9 ratio (0.8-1.2)
TT	13 secs (12-16.6 secs)
D-dimer	168ng/ml (<224ng/ml)
Fibrinogen	2.1g/dL (2-4g/dL)

- The patient has a normocytic anaemia.
- The prothrombin time (PT) is markedly deranged.

2) What is the likely cause of the clotting derangement? 1 mark

- Warfarin therapy.

3) How would you manage this patient? 4 marks

(1 mark for each correct stem)

- Acute assessment, resuscitation and management should be undertaken to follow an 'airway, breathing, circulation, disability and exposure' approach.
- Intravenous access and fluid resuscitation +/- blood transfusion.
- Mechanical and surgical attempts to stop the epistaxis.
- Correction of clotting.

4) How would you correct the clotting? 2 marks

(0.5 mark for each correct stem, with a maximum of 2 marks)

- Intravenous vitamin K.
- Fresh frozen plasma (FFP).
- Prothrombin complex concentrate.
- Recombinant factor VII.
- Discussion and advice from a haematologist.

5) How would you manage this patient's rib fractures? 1 mark

- These are usually managed conservatively.
- Analgesia is important to avoid complications such as basal atelectasis, a poor cough and poor clearance of secretions with potential pulmonary infection.

6) How would you manage this patient's pain? 2 marks

(0.5 mark for

- Simple analgesia (WHO analgesic ladder).
- Topical anaesthesia (lidocaine plasters).
- Regional anaesthesia (intercostal nerve blocks).
- Central neuroaxial anaesthesia (epidural, paravertebral blocks).

each correct

stem)

7) The patient goes to the ward and 4 days later 2 marks
you are called to see her. The Early Warning (0.5 mark for
Score is high and of note her heart rate is 120 each correct
bpm, the respiratory rate is 30 breaths per stem, with a
minute and her blood pressure is 75/40mmHg. maximum of 2
What are your differential diagnoses? marks)

- Bleed from intercostal vessels.
- Sepsis.
- Cardiac event.
- Anaemia.
- Further epistaxis.
- Pulmonary embolism.
- Other thromboembolic events (e.g. cerebrovascular event).

8) What investigations would you request?

- Bloods tests: full blood count, clotting, C-reactive 1 mark
protein (CRP).
- Chest X-ray. 0.5 mark
- Arterial blood gas. 0.5 mark

9) You are presented with the following chest X-ray (● Figure 5.5). Please comment on the significant abnormalities.

2 marks

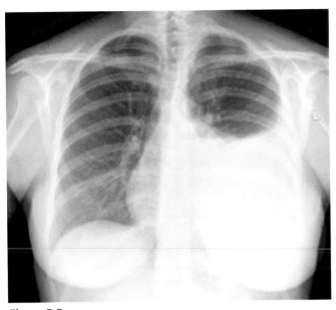

Figure 5.5.

There is a:

● Left-sided opacity in the lower zone, with a meniscus.
● Likely haemothorax.

10) What would be your specific management of this patient?

2 marks

(0.5 mark for each correct stem, with a maximum of 2 marks)

● Ensure clotting is corrected.
● Transfusion/fluid resuscitation.

- Intercostal drain.
- Interventional radiology for consideration of embolisation.
- Cardiothoracic surgical input, video-assisted thoracoscopic surgery (VATS).

References

1.   Ridley S, Taylor B, Gunning K. Medical management of bleeding in critically ill patients. *Cont Educ Anaesth Crit Care Pain* 2007; 7(4): 117.

Tumour lysis syndrome

A 43-year-old man presents to his family doctor with a progressive difficulty in breathing over the last few weeks. The patient is referred to the emergency department with acute respiratory failure and is investigated. He is subsequently diagnosed with acute lymphocytic leukaemia and is commenced on allopurinol, corticosteroids and has the first course of chemotherapy. Twelve hours later the patient is admitted to critical care.

1) Please summarise the blood tests below (●   2 marks Table 5.6).

Table 5.6. Blood test results.

Adjusted calcium	0.7mmol/L (2.2-2.6)
Na⁺	136mmol/L (136-148)
K⁺	6.9mmol/L (3.5-5.0)
Phosphate	2.36mmol/L (0.81-1.45)
Uric acid	748umol/L (200-430)
Glucose	6.6mmol/L (3.0-7.8)
CK	4000i.u./L (20-200)

- Hyperkalaemia, hyperuricaemia.
- Hyperphosphataemia, hypocalcaemia.

2) What is the most likely diagnosis? 1 mark

- Tumour lysis syndrome (TLS).

(Should the candidate fail to identify the diagnosis of tumour lysis syndrome, the examiner will inform the candidate of the diagnosis.)

3) What is the pathophysiology of tumour lysis syndrome?

2 marks
(1 mark for each correct stem, with a maximum of 2 marks)

- This is an oncological emergency due to a turnover of high cell mass malignancies resulting in severe metabolic derangement.
- TLS is an acute reaction to chemotherapy, radiotherapy or corticosteroids in lymphoproliferative malignancy.
- Usually it occurs 12-72 hours post-chemotherapy.

4) What are the risk factors for tumour lysis syndrome?

2 marks
(0.5 mark for each correct stem)

- Large tumour burden.
- Extensive bone marrow involvement.
- Leukaemias (all types), lymphomas (particularly Burkitt).
- Chemotherapy.

5) What other specific biochemical tests would you order and what would you expect to see?

2 marks

- Other renal biochemistry — raised urea and creatinine, in keeping with AKI.

- Arterial blood gas — metabolic acidosis; a low bicarbonate with hyperlactaemia.

6) What clinical features would you expect to see with tumour lysis syndrome?

3 marks (to include 5 clinical features)

- GI upset, fluid overload.
- Weakness, paraesthesia, tetany, hypocalcaemia.
- Arrhythmias — palpitations, chest pain, dyspnoea.
- Features of renal failure — oligoanuria, haematuria.

7) The candidate is shown an image (● Figure 5.6). Please present this radiological image and identify the key findings.

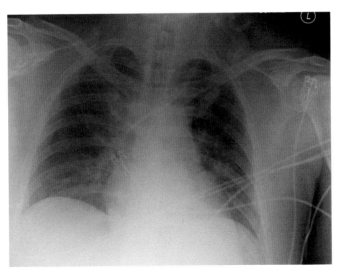

Figure 5.6.

- This is a chest radiograph — it is not apparent if it is 0.5 mark
PA or AP. There are no patient demographics. The
film is adequately penetrated and slightly rotated. The
trachea is central. There are ECG leads present.
- Widened mediastinum. 1 mark
- The right heart border is partly obscured. 0.5 mark
- A haemofiltration catheter, nasogastric tube and an 0.5 mark
endotracheal tube are *in situ*.
- Bilateral lung fields appear normal and the bony 0.5 mark
structures appear to be normal.

8) What are the preventative management measures? 2 marks

- Fluid optimised — well hydrated.
- Allopurinol.
- Monitor electrolytes.

9) What are the management strategies? 3 marks

Specific to TLS:

(1 mark for
each correct
stem, with a
maximum of 3
marks)

- Fluid resuscitation, diuretics.
- Management of electrolyte derangement:
  - hyperuricaemia:
    - xanthine oxidase inhibitors — allopurinol —
      inhibit uric acid formation;
    - urate oxidase or rasburicase — increase uric
      acid oxidation;
  - hyperkalaemia:
    - insulin and dextrose, salbutamol nebulizer —
      shift potassium intracellularly;
    - calcium gluconate — membrane stabilization;

- calcium resonium;
- hyperphosphataemia:
    - phosphate binders.
- replacement therapy.

References

1.   Beed M, Levitt M, Bokhari SW. Intensive care management of patients with haematological malignancy. *Cont Educ Anaesth Crit Care Pain* 2010; 10(6): 167-71.

Professionalism — omission of low-molecular-weight heparin

You are the doctor on-call for the ICU. The daughter of a patient on the unit has asked for an update on her father's condition. He was initially admitted following an emergency laparotomy 5 days ago. He went onto the ward but last night he became short of breath and started to complain of pleuritic chest pain. He had to be intubated on the ward and was transferred to the CT scanner where he was found to have a large pulmonary embolus. He is now stable on the ICU and his daughter has just been to visit him. On inspection of the patient's drug chart it appears that he was not prescribed low-molecular-weight heparin (LMWH). His daughter is unaware of this omission.

In this scenario the daughter will be played by an actor.

1) Please discuss the case with the daughter and outline the next steps.

The candidate:

- Provides an appropriate introduction, including their name, grade and role.   1 mark
- Establishes the identity of the patient's daughter and ensures she is the next of kin.   1 mark
- Outlines the events overnight to the daughter and answers any questions appropriately.   2 marks
- Informs the daughter of the diagnosis.   1 mark
- Informs the daughter that her father was not on LMWH.   1 mark

- Explains that it is likely that this contributed to the   1 mark
  pulmonary embolus.
- Apologises for the harm that has come to her father   1 mark
  due to this mistake.
- Avoids/explains 'jargon'.   1 mark
- Explains that this will be reported as a critical incident   6 marks
  and outlines the procedure for critical incident
  reporting:
  - critical incident reporting form;
  - this is forwarded to the manager/clinical lead for
    the ICU;
  - the incident is rated and is investigated;
  - the outcome of the investigation will be fed back
    to all stakeholders;
  - the principle is to identify areas where mistakes
    were made and put in processes to prevent
    further mistakes;
  - states that all patient safety issues are reported
    nationally via the National Reporting and
    Learning System (NRLS).
- Offers a further conversation with the consultant in   1 mark
  charge of the ICU.
- Suggests further areas of support, e.g. patient liaison   1 mark
  service.
- Closes the discussion appropriately.   1 mark
- Examiner to mark the candidate on whether they   2 marks
  communicated effectively.

Brainstem death testing

You are the doctor on the ICU and have been asked to carry out brainstem death testing on a 42-year-old man who sustained a catastrophic head injury following a road traffic accident.

There will be a manikin for the candidate to demonstrate the procedure.

1) **Before embarking on brainstem death testing, what criteria need to be fulfilled?**   3 marks

There must be evidence of:

- An apnoeic coma.
- A brain injury consistent with the clinical picture.
- All reversible causes of coma should be excluded, e.g. electrolytes, drugs, hypothermia.

2) **The candidate will then be asked to perform brainstem death testing on the manikin, talking through the process and the cranial nerves being tested.**

The following tests will be undertaken and the candidate must demonstrate the absence of the cranial nerve arc being tested.

- The caloric test assesses the cranial nerves (CN) VIII, CN III and CN VI.   1 mark
- Check the eardrum.   0.5 mark

- Irrigate the ear with 50ml of ice cold water whilst watching for nystagmus or deviation of the eyes.   0.5 mark
- Pupillary eye response assesses CN II and CN III, with both direct and consensual reflexes tested.   2 marks
- The corneal eye reflex assesses CN V and VII.   2 marks
- The gag reflex assesses CN IX and checks for any reaction to stimulation in the posterior pharynx.   1 mark
- The cough reflex assesses CN X and can be undertaken by suctioning via the endotracheal tube.   1 mark
- Painful stimuli applied to the supra-orbital ridge assesses CN VII, although grimacing to either central and peripheral stimulation, such as pressure over the nail bed, is acceptable as well.   2 marks

3) Please highlight the main points of the apnoea test.   3 marks

- Pre-oxygenate the patient for 5 minutes on 100% concentrated oxygen.
- Disconnect from the ventilator, and maintain oxygenation, e.g. with a suction catheter or apply 5cmH$_2$O of continuous positive airway pressure (CPAP) via a Mapleson C circuit.
- Observe for greater than 5 minutes or until PACO$_2$ >6.6kPa.

4) How quickly would you expect the PaCO$_2$ to rise?   1 mark

- 0.4-0.8kPa per minute.

5) How many times are the tests performed? 1 mark

- Two complete sets of brainstem death tests are required.

6) At what time is death confirmed? 1 mark

- At the end of the first set of tests.

7) Who can undertake the tests? 1 mark

- The consultant responsible for the patient's care.
- A second doctor who must be 5 years post-registration.

References

1. A code of practice for the diagnosis and confirmation of death. Academy of Medical Royal Colleges, 2008. http://www.bts.org.uk /Documents/A%20CODE%20OF%20PRACTICE%20FOR% 20THE%20DIAGNOSIS%20AND%20CONFIRMATION%20OF %20DEATH.pdf.

Abdominal compartment syndrome

A 62-year-old lady of Japanese descent was admitted to the hospital with jaundice and abdominal pain. The patient has been admitted under the care of general surgery with presumed obstructive gallstone-related pathology. Ultrasound of the abdomen has not revealed any gallstone pathology; however, the patient was found to have severe liver cirrhosis. The patient has developed a type I respiratory failure and is now hypotensive, tachycardic, tachypnoeic and febrile. The surgical team has requested a CT scan of the chest, abdomen and pelvis, and has asked for an intensive care review of the patient.

1) Describe the CT findings below (salient features only)(● Figure 5.7).   2 marks

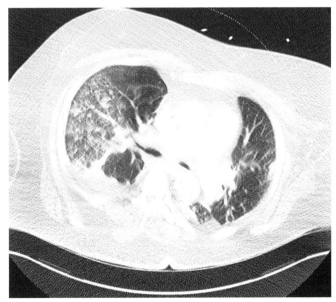

Figure 5.7.

- There is evidence of a bilateral ground-glass appearance, markedly seen on the right.
- Bilateral pleural effusions, the right larger than the left.

2) On review the patient has a distended abdomen which is moderately tender. There is a profound metabolic acidosis with a pH of 7.01, lactate of 6.1mmol/L and bicarbonate of 12mmol/L. On admission to intensive care the patient continues to have a raised lactate, is anuric, with a creatinine which doubles from 110μmol/l to 228μmol/l in a 24-hour period. What is the likely complication that has arisen? **1 mark**

- Abdominal compartment syndrome (ACS).

3) What is the normal intra-abdominal pressure (IAP)? **1 mark**

- Normal IAP = 5-7mmHg.

4) What is intra-abdominal hypertension (IAH)? **1 mark**

- IAP >12mmHg.

5) What is the definition of abdominal compartment syndrome? **2 marks**

- IAP >20mmHg.
- With new organ failure.

6) How would you classify ACS?

3 marks

(1 mark for each correct stem, with clear differentiation between the three)

- Primary ACS — an underlying injury such as a perforated bowel viscus or underlying intrabdominal disease causes ACS. This typically requires early surgical or radiological intervention.
- Secondary ACS — ACS is not due to a primary condition; for example, inflammation or capillary leak secondary to SIRS from acute pancreatitis.
- Recurrent ACS — ACS develops after previous surgical or medical treatment of ACS.

7) List some of the pathological sequelae as a result of ACS.

4 marks

(1 mark for each correctly named system and correct sub-stem describing the precise pathophysiology, with a maximum of 4 marks)

Multi-system effects:

- Respiratory effects:
  - elevation of the diaphragm;
  - reduced lung and chest wall compliance;
  - V/Q mismatch, hypoxia, hypercapnoea;
  - high inflation and plateau pressures.
- Renal:
  - compromised blood flow due to high intra-abdominal pressures;
  - decreased cardiac output causes a pre-renal insult;
  - subsequent compensatory increase in renal vascular resistance further compromises blood flow.
- Cardiovascular:
  - raised IAP causes direct compression of the inferior vena cava and portal vein;
  - preload is decreased as the increased intrathoracic pressure reduces venous return;

- cardiac compression and hence poor function;
- raised CVP.
- Neurological:
    - raised intracranial pressure.

8) What is the gold standard way of measuring   1 mark
IAP (● Figure 5.8)?

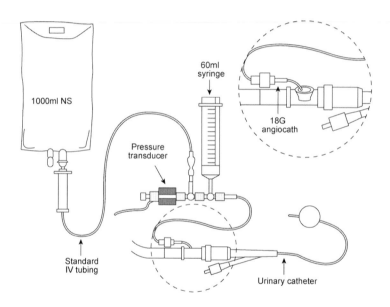

Figure 5.8.

- The gold standard method is using an intravesicular pressure measurement.

Top Tip

You may be given a diagram of the equipment used to measure IAP and asked to label it!

---

9) If the IAP is measured how would you relate this to the abdominal perfusion pressure?   1 mark

- APP = MAP - IAP.

  MAP — mean arterial pressure.

10) What are the management options for this patient with ACS?   4 marks
(1 mark for each correct stem, with a maximum of 4 marks)

- Optimising systemic perfusion and organ function through cautious fluid resuscitation and or vasopressor and inotrope administration may be necessary.
- Improving the abdominal wall compliance by enhancing sedation and analgesia may help — with or without muscle relaxation.
- Other measures include:
  - remove any restrictive dressings;
  - nasogastric decompression, prokinetics and enemas;

- the patient may benefit from diuretics and renal replacement therapy (RRT).
- If the IAP is not responding to these medical measures and remains sustained above 25mmHg then:
  - surgical decompression with a delayed closure may be necessary;
  - negative pressure dressings are recommended.

References

1. Cheatham ML, Malbrain ML, Kirkpatrick A, *et al*. Results from the International Conference of Experts in Intra-abdominal Hypertension and Abdominal Compartment Syndrome. II. Recommendations. *Intensive Care Med* 2007; 33: 951-62.

Dermatology — toxic epidermal necrolysis

A 56-year-old female with a background of being HTLV1-positive (human T-cell lymphotrophic virus 1) had been diagnosed a year previously with T-cell lymphoma. She had been successfully treated with the Newcastle Protocol of chemotherapy which had consisted of ifosfamide, etoposide and methotrexate. A recent CT showed no evidence of recurrent disease. The other notable comorbidities included Fanconi syndrome, chronic kidney disease with renal stones managed with a right JJ stent and notable malnutrition with a body mass index (BMI) of 17.

The patient has been admitted to hospital with urosepsis and has been commenced on intravenous ceftazidime and gentamicin. On day 3 of her admission she has a positive blood culture indicating an *Escherichia coli* bacteraemia. Microbiology doctors have advised to continue with intravenous ceftazidime. The patient has initially made improvements clinically, being more responsive, apyrexial and cardiovascularly stable.

1) Please study the results below in ● Table 5.7 and present the major findings.

2 marks
(1 mark for each correct stem, with a maximum of 2 marks)

Table 5.7. Blood test results.

	Day 1	Day 2	Day 3
Hb	120g/L	108g/L	106g/L
WCC	13.2 x 10^9/L	11.3 x 10^9/L	8.3 x 10^9/L
Platelets	39 x 10^9/L	30 x 10^9/L	21 x 10^9/L
Na$^+$	160mmol/L	149mmol/L	145mmol/L
Urea	8.8mmol/L	8.9mmol/L	7.7mmol/L
Creatinine	298μmol/L	287μmol/L	252μmol/L
CRP	157mg/L	196mg/L	167mg/L

- There is a mild anaemia and thrombocytopenia.
- With regards to the inflammatory markers, there is a fall in an initial raised WCC, but a plateau in the CRP.
- There is biochemical evidence of an acute kidney injury with an initially raised urea and creatinine.

2) However, by the eighth day of admission the patient was noted to have a blistering skin rash across her arms and upper torso. The rash was red, raised and appeared to peel away as layers in parts. Some portions had a blistering appearance. List some of the causes and differential diagnoses for these clinical developments.

3 marks
(1 mark for each correct stem, with a maximum of 3 marks)

- Systemic infective causes — bacterial (bacteraemia, septicaemia), for example, meningitis; viral, for example, a disseminated herpetic infection; protozoal or fungal.

- Cutaneous infective causes — cellulitis, necrotising fasciitis.
- Allergy, anaphylaxis or reaction to, for example, drugs such as antibiotics.
- Autoimmune, for example, bullous pemphigoid.
- Spectrum of toxic epidermal necrolysis and Stevens-Johnson syndrome.
- Nutritional deficit with cutaneous manifestation, for example, pellagra.

3) Of note is the severe pain associated with the affected areas. The patient deteriorates and the blistering rash starts to spread across the anterior and posterior aspects of the trunk, and the upper and lower limbs. The patient becomes oligoanuric. Interpret the physiological parameters and arterial blood gas in ● Table 5.8.

2 marks
(1 mark for each correct stem)

Table 5.8. Physiological parameters and arterial blood gas results.

BP	86/42mmHg
HR	119 bpm
Capillary refill time	4 seconds
pH	7.29
PaO_2	11.5kPa
$PaCO_2$	4.0kPa
HCO_3^-	21.1mmol/L
Lactate	3.9mmol/L
BE	-8.8mmol/L
Hb	92g/L

- The patient is tachycardic and hypotensive, with evidence of shock.
- There is a metabolic acidosis with attempted respiratory compensation, and a raised lactate.

4) What are the most likely diagnoses and what is the immediate management?

2 marks
(1 mark for each correct stem)

- A distributive shock likely to be due to:
  - sepsis;
  - a reaction to drugs — toxic epidermal necrolysis (TEN).
- The acute management should be assessment, resuscitation and management following an 'airway, breathing, circulation, disability and exposure' approach, the particular priority being fluid resuscitation.

5) A diagnosis of TEN is strongly suspected. How is this diagnosed?

1 mark
(all stems must be mentioned)

The diagnosis is made on:

- Clinical suspicion.
- Excluding other causes.
- Specific investigations to include a punch biopsy.

6) A dermatologist clinically diagnoses TEN with confirmation via a punch biopsy. List some precipitant causes of TEN and the most likely causes in this case.

3 marks
(1 mark for each correct stem, with a maximum of 3 marks)

- Malignancies such as lymphoma.

- Infections including viral, bacterial and protozoal sources.
- The most common precipitant factor for TEN is drug-induced.
- Drugs including cephalosporins, penicillins, quinolones, allopurinol, immunosuppressants and corticosteroids.
- In this case the cephalosporin and or infective source were suspected as the precipitant causes of the TEN.

7) On day 6 the TEN has spread to a body surface area of 70-80%. What are the specific management priorities for this patient with TEN and why?

6 marks
(1 mark for each correct stem and 3 marks for specific sub-stems)

The management can be thought of in three areas:

- The critical care supportive measures to include:
    - resuscitation and therapy following an 'airway, breathing, circulation, disability and exposure' protocol;
    - aggressive fluid resuscitation;
    - optimisation of nutritional state;
    - advanced cardiovascular monitoring;
    - multimodal analgesia.
- Specific measures for the TEN itself with removal or treatment of the precipitant cause, immunoglobulin (IVIg) therapy and possibly immunosuppressant therapy.

- Specialist care of the progressive cutaneous lesions can be thought of and managed as a severe extending burn injury:
  - warming and humidification of the environment;
  - vigilant management of the nutritional state due to a hypermetabolic state.

8) What is the prognosis for this patient and how can this be guided?

1 mark
(0.5 mark for each correct stem)

- The prognosis is poor with a mortality associated with TEN to be greater than 58%.
- The prognosis can be guided by a TEN severity of illness scale called the SCORTEN scale.

Top Tip

TEN has a severity of illness scale called the SCORTEN scale [1]. The score estimates the mortality of TEN by looking at seven variables as listed below (● Table 5.9). In this particular case, the mortality from TEN was predicted at 58.6%. This illustrates the severity of the condition. This patient has other comorbidities which make the prognosis very poor as the TEN progressively worsened.

Table 5.9. SCORTEN scale — risk factors.

Risk factor	0	1
Age	<40 years	>40 years
Associated malignancy	No	Yes
Heart rate (beats/min)	<120	>120
Serum BUN (mg/dL)	<27	>27
Detached or compromised body surface	<10%	>10%
Serum bicarbonate (mEq/L)	>20	<20
Serum glucose (mg/dL)	<250	>250

The reaction to the drug may have a latent period of up to 21 days. Presentation can initially be progressive with a subsequent rapid course. The patient can experience a painful and burning rash with mucosal involvement. On examination the patient will have target lesions, with mucocutaneous vesicles and papules.

Management of the patient with TEN is largely supportive and determined by the severity. The critical care environment is important in more severe cases involving a total body surface area of >30%, as the patient will require large fluid volume resuscitation, advanced cardiovascular monitoring, multimodal analgesia and careful nursing. Isolation to decrease superimposed infection is important. Reverse barrier nurse management will further help with this. The care of the cutaneous lesions will be similar to a patient with extensive burns. As with burns victims there is a hypermetabolic state and, hence, optimised nutrition is important. This may be through early calorific enteral feeding and vigilant monitoring of nutritional state. Warming and humidification of the environment can be important measures [2].

Specific management with IVIg has been explored over a number of trials. French *et al* looked at these trials and reported that 6 out of the 8 studies had indicated a decrease in mortality with IVIg at doses of greater than 2g/kg [3]. The role of steroids, however, is more contentious as there is a proposed increased risk of infection [2].

References

1. Bastuji-Garin S, Fouchard N, Bertocchi M, *et al.* SCORTEN: a severity-of-illness score for toxic epidermal necrolysis. *J Invest Dermatol* 2000; 115: 149-53.

2. Ghislain PD, Roujeau JC. Treatment of severe drug reactions: Stevens-Johnson syndrome, toxic epidermal necrolysis and hypersensitivity syndrome. *Dermatol Online J* 2002; 8(1): 5.

3. French LE, Trent JT, Francisco AK. Use of intravenous immunoglobulin in toxic epidermal necrolysis and Stevens-Johnson syndrome: our current understanding. *Int Immunopharmacol* 2006; 6(4): 543-9.

Viral haemorrhagic fever — Ebola

A 48-year-old male is brought into the emergency department by ambulance after suffering a seizure at home. He is now 9/15 on the Glasgow Coma Scale (GCS) and is being stabilised prior to being taken for a CT scan of his head. The patient has recently returned from Liberia. He has the following physiological recordings:

- Heart rate — 119 beats per minute.
- Blood pressure — 82/48mmHg.
- Temperature — 42°C.

1) An arterial blood gas (ABG) has been performed (Table 5.10). Please summarise the results.

2 marks

Table 5.10. Arterial blood gas results.	
pH	7.19
PaO_2	14.4kPa
$PaCO_2$	3.7kPa
HCO_3^-	19.6mmol/L
Lactate	5.6mmol/L
BE	-8mmol/L

- There is a metabolic acidosis and lactataemia.
- With attempted respiratory compensation.

2) Some of the salient blood results are listed below in ● Table 5.11. What are the main problems with his physiological parameters and blood results?

3 marks
(1 mark for each correct stem, with a maximum of 3 marks)

Table 5.11. Blood test results.

Hb	100g/L
WCC	2.4×10^9/L
Platelets	110×10^9/L
INR	1.9
Na$^+$	135mmol/L
K$^+$	4.9mmol/L
HCO$_3^-$	18mmol/L
Urea	13.0mmol/L
Creatinine	167µmol/L
The D-dimer	Raised

- Tachycardia, hypotension, fever with a low conscious state.
- Pancytopenia — anaemia, thrombocytopaenia, low white cell count (WCC).
- Acute kidney injury — raised urea and creatinine.
- The INR is deranged — potential coagulopathy.

3) His wife tells you that he has been generally unwell since returning from Liberia 4 days ago with progressively worsening diarrhoea, vomiting and severe abdominal cramps in the last 2 days. Associated with this he has had a fever, cough and headache.

4 marks

Given this history and recent foreign travel what potential diagnoses would you be vigilant to?

- Malaria.
- Gram-negative septic shock.
- Viral haemorrhagic fever (VHF) — Ebola.
- Thrombotic thrombocytopenic purpura (TTP).

4) What other clinical feature would you ask about or look for in this patient which may help distinguish viral haemorrhagic fever?   1 mark

A recent development of the following features would be indicative of VHF over malaria:

- Extensive bruising.
- Active bleeding.

Top Tip

In this case the central nervous symptomology with seizures bring all four of these differentials into play, for example, cerebral malaria, febrile seizures secondary to sepsis, meningitis, encephalitis or the central nervous system sequelae from TTP. Some further details on Ebola are provided below.

293

5) If Ebola as well as malaria and septic shock were all potentially suspected, what are the main principles of management for this patient?

10 marks
(1 mark for each correct stem)

This patient should be managed with vigilance towards infective conditions including Ebola, malaria and septic shock from potentially bacterial meningitis. A high degree of suspicion is necessary for all three. Management generically should include:

- Acute assessment, resuscitation and management should be undertaken to follow an 'airway, breathing, circulation, disability and exposure' approach.
- Isolation, with limitation of the number of staff and family exposed to the patient.
- Escalation to the named consultant and nursing coordinator for a suspected case of Ebola.
- Escalation to the named on-call public health lead for the hospital which may be the on-call microbiologist or infectious diseases consultant.
- In the meantime specific management for septic shock, meningitis and potentially malaria should be commenced.

Management highlights specific to viral haemorrhagic fever should include:

- Referral to the named Ebola specialist centre.
- Isolation, ideally in a negative pressure room.
- Specialist tests for Ebola:
  - antigen-capture enzyme-linked immunosorbent assay (ELISA) testing;
  - IgM ELISA;
  - polymerase chain reaction (PCR);
  - virus isolation.

- Specific tests to rule out other differentials, for example, malaria.
- Public health referral.

Top Tip

Ebola has become a devastating outbreak primarily affecting Sierra Leone, Guinea, Nigeria and Liberia. Although this presentation above has been few and far between, it could yet be a potential hazard facing all hospitals.

Ebola is a RNA flavivirus causing VHF. It has a related symptomology to yellow fever, Lassa fever and dengue fever. Its primary reservoir is believed to be in fruit bats, but human consumption of these fruit bats or non-human primates who may have consumed the fruit bats is the postulated theory of transfer. The transmission is through direct body fluids including blood, saliva, faeces, urine and sweat. These fluids need to transmit from the infected individual through the new host's mucous membranes or broken skin.

The symptomology includes:

- Severe gastroenterological features such as diarrhoea, vomiting and abdominal cramps.
- Features of a consumptive coagulopathy with bleeding and/or bruising.

- Generalised symptomology of fever, malaise and headache.
- Features of septic shock.

The features above are very non-specific, hence the diagnosis must be attached to a high index of suspicion married up with the history. These patients will develop multi-organ failure and can rapidly deteriorate. Whilst this is important, the Ebola-positive casualty also poses a potent threat to everyone in close contact.

Personal protective equipment is mandated and crucial in the care of Ebola victims and prevention of spread. The suspicion of this condition is a critical notifiable condition. There should be a clearly documented pathway with named experts within the hospital to engage with the correct escalation and reporting, in this case to Public Health England with urgent transfer to the Royal Free Hospital in London for specialist Ebola isolation and care.

The United Kingdom government has released comprehensive guidance on the management of a suspected case of VHF. The following web site has regular updated versions on the guidance for Ebola and VHF:

https://www.gov.uk/government/publications/viral-haemorrhagic-fever-algorithm-and-guidance-on-management-of-patients.

Index

M

macrolides 162

malignant disease

    disseminated 95-8

    tumour lysis syndrome 267-71

medical errors

    critical incident reporting 31-2

    failure to prescribe heparin 272-3

    NG tube misplacement 187-9, 211-12

meningitis 104

microbiology

    Guillain-Barré syndrome 48

    necrotising fasciitis 135

    pneumonia 42-3, 161-2

    sepsis 207

middle cerebral artery (MCA) infarcts 58-9

mitral stenosis 202

muscle injury (rhabdomyolysis) 181-6

muscular spasms (tetanus) 226-9

myasthenia gravis 125-8

myocardial infarction 77-81, 110-11, 233-4

myocardial ischaemia 171-2

N

nasogastric (NG) tube misplacement 187-9, 211-12

National Institutes of Health Stroke Scale (NIHSS) 248

neck injury 176-7

necrotising fasciitis 133-7

nosocomial pneumonia 43

nutrition, refeeding syndrome 212-14

O

oesophageal Doppler 11, 90

oesophageal varices 230-2

osmolality 19, 216